Guide to Interpreting
Spectral Domain
Optical Coherence Tomography

D0907558

Guide to Interpreting Spectral Domain Optical Coherence Tomography

SECOND EDITION

Bruno Lumbroso MD
Centro Oftalmologico Mediterraneo
Via Brofferio 7
Rome, Italy
Bruno.lumbroso@gmail.com

Marco Rispoli MD
Centro Oftalmologico Mediterraneo
Via Brofferio 7
Rome, Italy

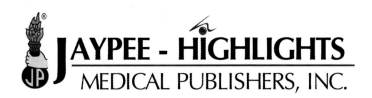

JAYPEE - HIGHLIGHTS
MEDICAL PUBLISHERS, INC.

Published by

Jaypee Brothers Medical Publishers (P) Ltd

Corporate Office

4838/24 Ansari Road, Daryaganj, **New Delhi** - 110002, India
Phone: +91-11-43574357, Fax: +91-11-43574314
Website : www.jaypeebrothers.com

Offices in India

- **Ahmedabad**, e-mail: ahmedabad@jaypeebrothers.com
- **Bengaluru**, e-mail: bangalore@jaypeebrothers.com
- **Chennai**, e-mail: chennai@jaypeebrothers.com
- **Delhi**, e-mail: jaypee@jaypeebrothers.com
- **Hyderabad**, e-mail: hyderabad@jaypeebrothers.com
- **Kochi**, e-mail: kochi@jaypeebrothers.com
- **Kolkata**, e-mail: kolkata@jaypeebrothers.com
- **Lucknow**, e-mail: lucknow@jaypeebrothers.com
- **Mumbai**, e-mail: mumbai@jaypeebrothers.com
- **Nagpur**, e-mail: nagpur@jaypeebrothers.com

Overseas Offices

- **Central America Office, Panama City, Panama,** Ph: 001-507-317-0160
  e-mail: cservice@jphmedical.com,   Website: www.jphmedical.com
- **Europe Office, UK,** Ph: +44 (0) 2031708910
  e-mail: info@jpmedpub.com

Guide to Interpreting Spectral Domain Optical Coherence Tomography

© 2011, Jaypee Brothers Medical Publishers

All rights reserved. No part of this publication should be reproduced, stored in a retrieval system, or transmitted in any form or by any means: electronic, mechanical, photocopying, recording, or otherwise, without the prior written permission of the authors and the publisher.

This book has been published in good faith that the material provided by authors is original. Every effort is made to ensure accuracy of material, but the publisher, printer and authors will not be held responsible for any inadvertent error(s). In case of any dispute, all legal matters to be settled under Delhi jurisdiction only.

Second Edition: **2011**

ISBN 978-93-5025-384-7

Printed in India

Preface to the Second Edition

The purpose of this book is to help optical coherence tomography (OCT) users interpret images that, at the beginning, may look very complex and bewildering. We use a logical method for interpreting OCT images. The first phase of analysis subdivides each image into its smallest components. The second phase combines these fine details to arrive at a synthesis; from then, to an accurate diagnosis and decide an appropriate therapy.

This manual features detailed schematic illustrations as well as actual scans, and is a step-by-step guide for interpreting images acquired by spectral domain OCT. It gives information on technical and clinical possibilities in the study of glaucoma and on three-dimensional images.

We intend to help the readers reach logical interpretations of the OCT scans and assist OCT users in the difficult task of sifting through the mass of data to extract useful information.

Originally written for OCT Zeiss Cirrus users, it has been modified, thanks to Jaypee Brothers Medical Publishers, to be offered to a wider audience. We thank Zeiss executives who urged and assisted us in writing a basic OCT guidebook, and Jaypee Brothers Medical Publishers who proposed to modify it for a wider group of users.

Bruno Lumbroso
Marco Rispoli

Contents

PART ONE

INTRODUCTION

Optical coherence tomography (OCT) is an essential tool for diagnosing and managing retinal diseases and glaucoma. In this handbook, which features detailed schematic illustrations as well as actual OCT scans, we offer a step-by-step guide for interpreting images and data acquired by the revolutionary and novel spectral domain OCT technology.

We believe this handbook is important because spectral domain technology offers significant advances over time domain technology. For example, spectral domain OCT offers:

1. Improvements to the sagittal OCT B-scan, which reveals previously undetected structures
2. Technical and clinical improvements in the study of glaucoma
3. Three-dimensional images that provide new information. (Although this is a new way to view ocular structures, interpretation can be learned quickly and easily, and these images enable more accurate diagnosis.)

All references to spectral domain OCT in this handbook are based on our experiences with the spectral domain Cirrus™ HD-OCT manufactured by Carl Zeiss Meditec Inc., Dublin, Calif. (U.S. headquarters). All images were generated by the Cirrus™ HD-OCT.

In these pages, we have ascribed great importance to explaining the meaning of OCT images. In addition, we have tried to set forth a logical method for interpreting ophthalmic images. The first phase of analysis subdivides each image into its smallest components. The second phase combines these fine details to synthesize the data, enabling us to arrive at an accurate diagnosis and to decide on appropriate therapy. We hope this handbook helps eyecare practitioners appreciate the new possibilities offered by spectral domain OCT.

Bruno Lumbroso
Marco Rispoli

Chapter 1

Overview of Optical Coherence Tomography

Advances in technology usher in a new era of expanded functionality.

Optical coherence tomography (OCT) is an essential tool for noninvasive *in vivo* analysis of retinal tissue for diagnosis and management of retinal disease and glaucoma. This technique is based on the degree of absorption or dispersion of light traversing the tissue. The light, which is divided into a detection arm and a reference arm, is emitted by a superluminescent diode at a wavelength of approximately 840 nm.

Time domain OCT, which was commercialized at the end of 1996 and improved with increased resolution in 2002, compares a reflected beam of light to a beam of light from a reference mirror. Time

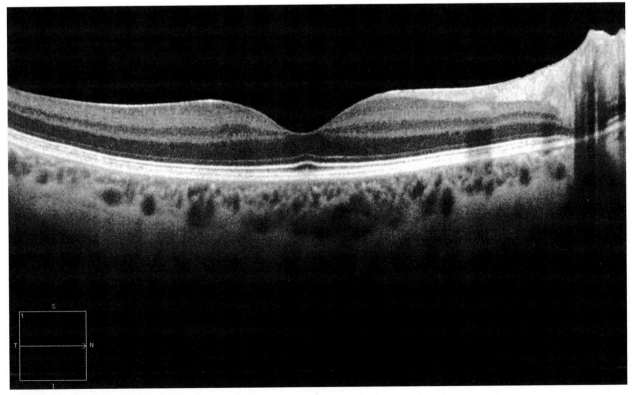

FIGURE 1.
Cirrus™ HD-OCT image of a healthy retina. Courtesy of David S. Boyer, M.D.

delays between the two beams can then be measured. Although the low acquisition rate exposes the images to aberrations caused by eye movement, increasing the acquisition speed would degrade image resolution. At good resolution (1024 points in 6 mm of tissue), time domain OCT can produce one B-scan every 1.6 seconds (400 A-scans per second).

SPECTRAL DOMAIN OCT

Recently, we have seen the emergence of a new technology called Fourier domain or spectral domain OCT, which employs a different acquisition technique. This technique uses a spectrometer on the detector arm to measure the difference in wavelength between the light from the fixed reference arm and that returning from the tissue. The instrument uses Fourier analysis to analyze the images according to the light wavelength recorded.

This type of OCT technology avoids moving the reference arm and instead analyzes the reflected light using a spectrometer. The immediate advantage of this technology is the high number of scans acquired per second—approximately 27,000 A-scans per second-making true three-dimensional (3-D) imaging possible and practical in a clinial environment.

This sampling frequency has notable advantages. The possibility of artifacts due to eye movement is minimized because the operator can easily position and center the beam to control the image, especially when working with pseudophakic or highly myopic eyes, or when there is relevant media opacity. Given the increased resolution, fine retinal detail is comparable to what is visible on a histology slide.

The Cirrus™ HD-OCT combines image accuracy and ease of use. The acquisition process is fully automated, including:

- Auto focus
- Auto optimization
- Auto polarization.

Cycles follow one another in a few seconds, placing the retinal plane in the center of the screen. The operator need only position the scanner on the area of the retina to be studied. The instrument acquires in high-resolution or high-speed mode, taking into consideration the inverse proportions between these variables.

As mentioned previously, the wavelength of the light source is 840 nm, and the sampling frequency is about 27,000 A-scans per second. The instrument acquires 200 to 512 B-scans in rapid succession, from top to bottom, then constructs a 3-D retinal map by aligning the B-scans. Acquisition speed determines the accuracy of the retinal map, so with spectral domain technology, it is possible to obtain very detailed retinal maps.

The analysis speed for calculation of average thickness and the display of ETDRS grid averages is almost the same. The higher density of data collected with spectral domain technology also allows for 3-D display.

Chapter 2

General Principles for Obtaining and Interpreting Spectral Domain OCT Images

Compared with time domain OCT, spectral domain OCT provides more detailed images and more data with improved speed and accuracy for in-depth analysis.

Spectral domain optical coherence tomography (SD-OCT) allows us to visualize cross-sectional, anterior segment, and three-dimensional (3-D) views of the retina. This enables us to diagnose glaucoma and retinal diseases and monitor treatment efficacy. The data provided by SD-OCT are analogous to those obtained with ultrasound B examinations, but with some notable advantages. For example, the resolution of ultrasound B is about 150 microns, while the resolution of time domain OCT is 10 microns, and the resolution of SD-OCT is 5 microns.

Retinal scans with SD-OCT are highly reproducible. A few trace points on the margin of the optic nerve or the retinal vasculature allow the registration of one scan to another. In addition, the instrument is easy to operate.

Optical coherence tomography allows clinical observation, measurement, and identification of structures that otherwise are not easily visible, such as the external limiting membrane (ELM) and the junction between the internal and external segment of the photoreceptors (IS/OS junction). It also shows various types of lesions with altered morphology, altered reflectivity and/or optically blank areas. OCT performs the following functions:

- Measures retinal thickness
- Measures the retinal nerve fiber layer (RNFL)
- Measures the volume of the retina
- Creates retinal thickness maps
- Isolates and creates maps of the internal limiting membrane (ILM) and the retinal pigment epithelium (RPE)
- Measures various parameters of the optic disc
- Displays three-dimensional views
- Provides classic C-scan (*en-face*) analyses, creating horizontal tissue sections
- Offers an RPE-fit function, which provides a view of a tissue section.

The images obtained can be analyzed, quantified, saved, compared with other results, and superimposed on fluorescein angiography, indocyanine green, and microperimetry.

Spectral domain OCT is a reliable and sensitive examination. The images are reproducible. Scan acquisition is rapid and simple, and does not require the administration of intravenous contrast media. In some cases, such as retinal edema follow-up, OCT may be preferable to fluorescein angiography, which is an invasive test that may lead to complications.

OBTAINING OPTIMAL OCT IMAGES

The most frequent impediments to acquiring good OCT images are ocular movement, media opacity, and an uncooperative patient. Images taken through miotic pupils are generally good. In rare cases, dilation of the pupils is necessary. A normal lacrimal film or good corneal hydration with artificial tears is necessary. Although it is possible to obtain images when early cataracts are present or when intraocular silicone oil is present, these conditions may interfere with scan quality. The following tips may help you obtain optimal OCT images.

GENERAL

Corneal conditions can affect the clarity of an OCT image and, therefore, may interfere with accurate interpretation. A dry eye, especially in the elderly, can lead to greatly compromised images. In these cases, it is best to instill artificial tears before the OCT examination.

Acquisitions with SD-OCT instruments can sometimes produce artifacts. Artifacts are often caused by poor fixation or lack of cooperation by the patient, including excessive blinking. The patient should fixate on the stimulus — a cross of green segments similar to a star — in the interior of the instrument's optics. During the examination, the patient can see the stimulus and the red scanning segment at the same time, which may distract the patient, especially if the visual acuity is good.

These intrinsic and extrinsic factors may cause artifacts to a greater or lesser degree, depending on the type of acquisition protocol.

5-LINE RASTER

Usually, this test is less affected by ocular movement because scanning time is relatively short. The most frequent artifact is a shading or, more precisely, a portion of the scan showing an offset of the pixels on the horizontal axis that is distinct from the "granular" pixelation display of the rest of the B-scan.

MACULAR CUBE 512X128

For this type of acquisition, the patient must fixate on the target for 2.4 seconds. During the scan, the screen shows the operator an external view of the eye, a real-time fundus image, OCT images of the central crosshair, and the top and bottom B-scans. After capture, the "Review" screen provides qualitative information on the scan. If a patient blinks during the scan, the horizontal segments will appear black on the OCT image. If a patient loses fixation, saccades will be present where the blood vessels are not contiguous. If blinks or numerous artifacts are present, the operator clicks the "Try Again" button to return to the "Scan Acquisition" screen.

TABLE 1: CAPABILITIES OF SD-OCT
In our experience, spectral domain optical coherence tomography (SD-OCT) offers the following advantages: • Simple, with a short learning curve • Fast (2.4 seconds or less) • Reliable • Sensitive (resolution of 5 microns) • Reproducible • Noninvasive, noncontact and safe **With SD-OCT, clinicians can:** • Detect disease • Evaluate treatment efficacy over time • Quantify lesion thickness and volume • Track disease progression • Evaluate postoperative status • Study 3D views **Conditions that can affect the quality of OCT scans include:** • Transparency of the optic media • Poor corneal condition or lacrimal film

Interpreting the Complete Image: Analysis and Synthesis

Even before we began our study of medicine, we learned that in order to decipher various data in science, we must apply a logical method according to coherent criteria. Studying a complete image to obtain a diagnosis and thus formulate a therapeutic decision is not a simple process. The logical method is divided into two parts: the analysis, which further divides each argument or image into its constituent elements, and the synthesis, which then reunites the elements that were isolated.

A logical method underlies evidence-based medicine and should be applied in all of our activities as clinicians, including OCT analysis. Reading an OCT report involves:

- *Qualitative, 2D, and 3D images and maps*
- *Quantitative analytical tests: retinal thickness, retinal map, volumetry*
- *Synthesis of all examination findings, including retinal thickness, morphological alterations, hyper- and hypo-reflectivity, and anomalous structures apparent with fluorescein and indocyanine green.*

Using this information, we can reach a diagnosis.

René Descartes, the 17th-century French philosopher, elucidated the principles of analysis and synthesis in "Le Discours de la Mèthode" in 1637, which stated:

The science of the intellect is universal, and there can only be one true method, which consists of separating what is already simple and clear in order then to attempt to understand that which is complex and obscure. The method is a collection of reliable, easy rules, observing which there is no risk of mistaking the false for the true.

In a logical process, the analyses of each of the possible elements is first performed: Then after this phase, the synthesis of all these elements is performed, and the results of these flow into the conclusions.

To replace the apparent chaos of data with an ordered and rationally constructed system.

Chapter 3

Interpretation of Pathological Cross-sectional OCT

In this chapter, we discuss how to interpret the two-dimensional cross-sectional spectral domain OCT scan, the B-scan.

Following a logical sequence is essential when analyzing an optical coherence tomography (OCT) scan. Initially, each of the elements - hyperreflective lesions, hyporeflective lesions, anatomical changes, quantitative alterations, retinal thickness, and retinal map - must be analyzed to arrive at an interpretation.

INTERPRETING COLORS ON SPECTRAL DOMAIN OCT

Generally, it is preferable to study images in gray scale instead of conventional pseudo colors. This allows us to evaluate slight variations in the intensities of gray to distinguish details that are easy to miss.

TABLE 1: ANALYSIS AND SYNTHESIS USING OCT

I. ANALYTIC STUDY

QUALITATIVE ANALYSIS

A. MORPHOLOGY

Morphological alterations
- Deformation of the entire retina
- Alteration of the retinal profile
- Intraretinal structural alteration
- Morphological alteration of the posterior layer

Anomalous structures
- Preretinal
- Epiretinal
- Intraretinal
- Subretinal

3-D and C-scan studies
- Cystoid edema
- Serous RPE detachment
- Serous neuroepithelium detachment
- Neovascular membrane
- Lamellar hole
- Macular hole

B. REFLECTIVITY

Increased reflectivity
- Superficial
- Intraretinal
- Deep

Decreased reflectivity
- Superficial
- Intraretinal
- Deep

Shadow zones – screen effect
- Anterior
- Superficial
- Deep

QUANTITATIVE ANALYSIS
- Thickness
- Volume
- Map

II. SYNTHESIS
By evaluating and comparing OCT data in conjunction with the patient's history, the clinical examination and other tests, clinicians can arrive at a diagnosis or evaluate the patient's response to therapy.

The spectral domain OCT (SD-OCT) software arbitrarily assigns a color for each degree of reflectivity, allowing us to see marked differences in color where we would otherwise observe a gradual change in reflectivity **(Figures 1, 2).**

QUALITATIVE ANALYSIS: MORPHOLOGY

Compared with time domain OCT, SD-OCT instruments offer a clearer and more detailed view of pathology throughout the entire retina. With

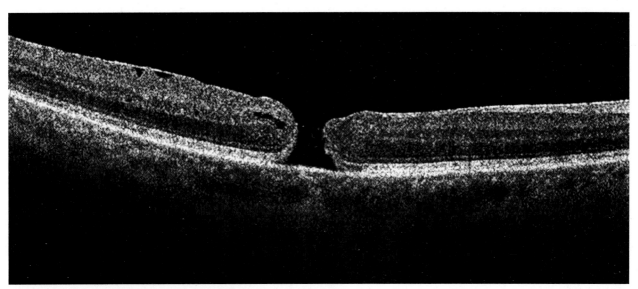

FIGURE 1. PATHOLOGICAL IMAGE IN GRAY SCALE.

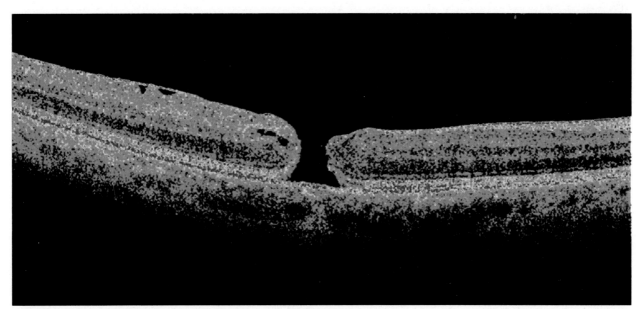

FIGURE 2. PATHOLOGICAL IMAGE IN COLOR SCALE.
Special domain OCT software automatically selects the level of reflectivity to attribute to a certain color, which can be particularly helpful in teaching or in discussions with patients. In the full-thickness macular hole shown above on gray scale, the ELM is much clearer and easier to observe, and the RPE appears clearly subdivided into three layers. With the color scale, these details are difficult to see.

SD-OCT, retinal layers, particularly the external retina, the photoreceptors, and the retinal pigment epithelium (RPE), can be differentiated, and morphological variations can be evaluated. Subtle histological structures, which may be missed with time domain OCT, can be detected with SD-OCT.

In addition, SD-OCT can discern the intravitreal formations, strands, and particles that may be found in inflammation, hemorrhage, or neovascularization. The vitreoretinal interface and hyaloid are also more visible with SD-OCT.

RETINAL DEFORMATIONS

- *Concavity (myopia):* In cases of high myopia **(Figure 3)** and especially posterior myopic staphyloma **(Figure 4)**, OCT will show a marked concavity. Certain lesions in the sclera (staphylomas) contribute to a localized depression of the retina throughout its thickness.

- *Convexity (cysts or subretinal tumors):* In cases of serous detachment of the RPE, OCT often shows a convex shape. In rare instances, however, convexity may be due to subretinal cysts. In these

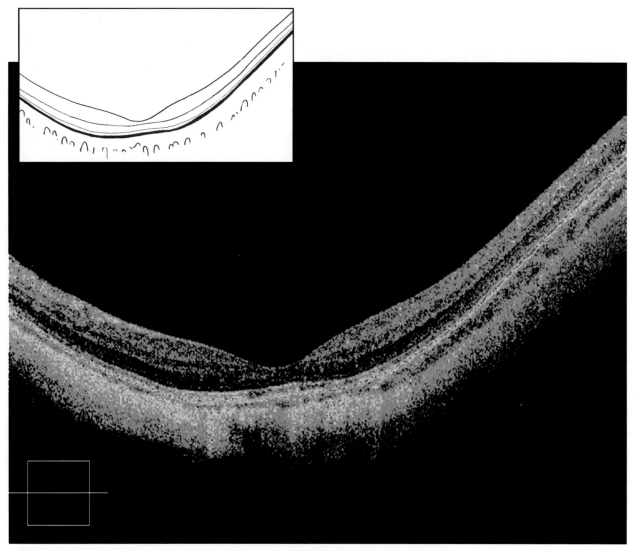

FIGURE 3. QUALITATIVE ANALYSIS – MORPHOLOGY – DEFORMATION OF THE ENTIRE RETINA.
Note the abnormally concave structure of this highly myopic eye (21 diopters).

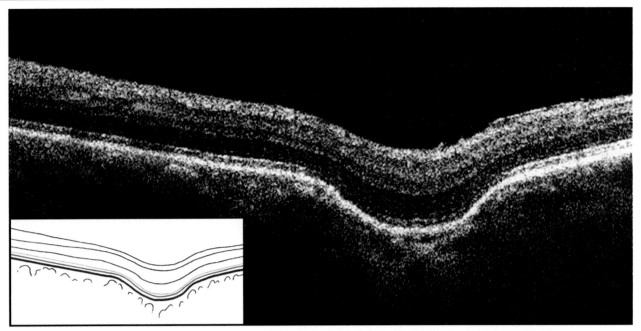

FIGURE 4. QUALITATIVE ANALYSIS – MORPHOLOGY – DEFORMATION OF THE ENTIRE RETINA – SMALL STAPHYLOMA.
This is a rare case of a small posterior staphyloma of the retina due to a localized deformation of the sclera from possible scleritis. The retina is preserved over all layers and follows the scleral deformation without changing its structure.

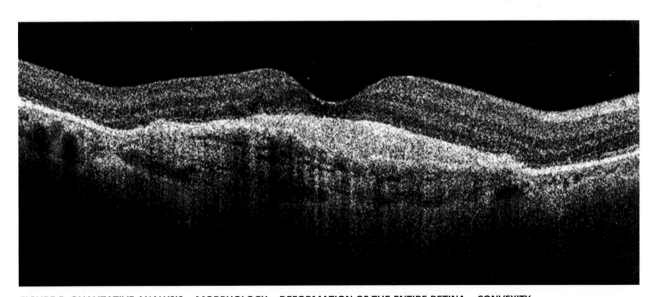

FIGURE 5. QUALITATIVE ANALYSIS – MORPHOLOGY – DEFORMATION OF THE ENTIRE RETINA – CONVEXITY.
In cases of subretinal cysts or choroidal tumors, a convex retina that also involves the RPE and the choriocapillaris may be observed. In this case of fibrovascular scarring and neovascularization, retinal edema and small serous detachments of the retina are seen. The retina is deformed and convex.

cases, the convexity is less pronounced and includes the subretinal layers (the epithelium and choriocapillaris). In subretinal tumors, such as melanomas, the entire retina, including the RPE, may be raised and differentiating the tumor may be difficult **(Figure 5)**.

ABNORMAL RETINAL PROFILE

The normal retinal profile shows a regular, symmetrical foveal depression. Optical coherence tomography can detect abnormalities, such as:

- *Vitreoretinal traction.* The normal foveal depression deforms, becoming convex and/or irregular. This condition is associated with the formation of fissures or holes **(Figure 6)**.
- *Diffuse retinal edema.* The foveal depression may be reduced or disappear, and the retinal profile may become flat or slightly irregular. The absence of the foveal depression is a sign of clinically significant retinal edema.
- *Complex vitreoretinal traction.*
- *Retinal folds*
- *Macular pucker.* The retinal surface is deformed by waves and curled by traction caused by the epiretinal membrane (ERM) **(Figures 7, 8)**.

TABLE 1: RETINAL PROFILES SEEN WITH SD-OCT

- Normal profile
- Enlarged foveal depression
- Decreased foveal depression
- Asymmetric foveal depression
- Absent foveal depression
- Retinal convexity from edema or traction instead of the depression
- Profile deformed by localized vitreoretinal traction
- Profile deformed by complex vitreoretinal traction
- Retinal profile undulating due to retinal folds
- Retinal profile corrugated due to narrow retinal folds
- Retinal convexity from edema or traction instead of the depression
- Macular hole
- Lamellar hole
- Macular pucker

ENLARGED AND IRREGULAR FOVEAL DEPRESSION

Macular Pseudohole

An enlarged foveal depression simulates a retinal macular hole. The presence of tissue at all retinal layers above the RPE is a pseudohole. A true lamellar hole is characterized by an absence of some retinal layers above the RPE **(Figure 9)**.

Macular Hole

Optical coherence tomography facilitates identification, measurement, and classification of macular holes according to the Gass classifications. The C-scan or RPE-fit view allows qualitative evaluation of edema, if present.

- *Stage 1:* The foveal depression disappears, and a small optically blank area (cyst) forms below the retinal surface **(Figure 10)**.
- *Stage 2:* Partial breaks of the internal retina are apparent, with operculum adhering to the margins of the hole, and slightly increased thickness.
- *Stage 3:* The hole's full-thickness operculum is no longer adherent to the retina. Retinal edema may be present, with increased thickness of the retina and a small detachment.

TABLE 2: FEATURES SEEN WITH SD-OCT

Anomalous structures

INTERNAL RETINA
- Vitreoretinal interface abnormalities
- Preretinal and peripapillary neovascular membranes
- Preretinal or epiretinal membrane

EXTERNAL RETINA
- Exudates
- Drusen
- Neovascular membranes
  - Classic lesion
  - Occult lesion
  - Macular scar

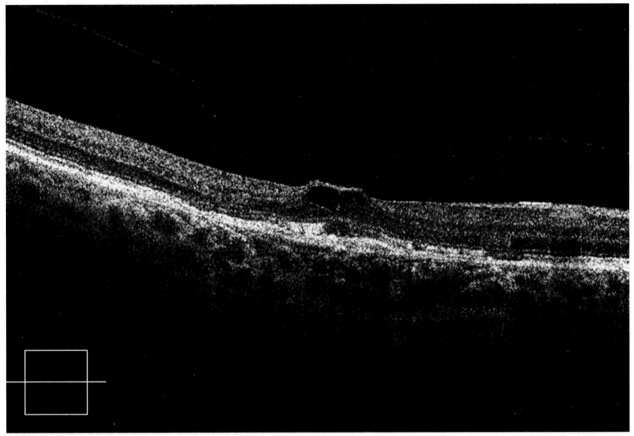

FIGURE 6. QUALITATIVE ANALYSIS – MORPHOLOGY – DEFORMATION OF THE RETINAL PROFILE FROM LOCALIZED VITREORETINAL TRACTION.
Partially adherent epiretinal membrane exerts traction on the retinal surface, causing the foveal depression to disappear. An intraretinal cyst forms at the localized traction.

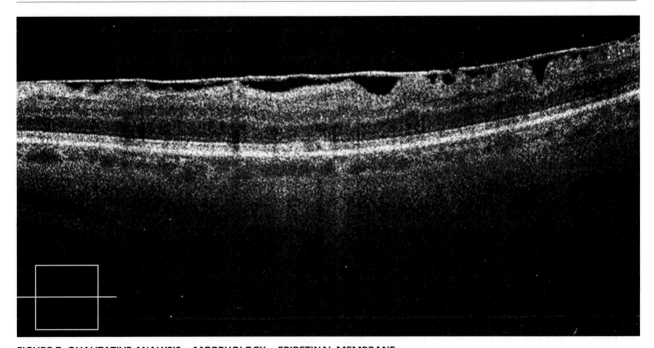

FIGURE 7. QUALITATIVE ANALYSIS – MORPHOLOGY – EPIRETINAL MEMBRANE.
Partially adherent epiretinal membrane exerts tangential traction on the retinal surface, causing folds on the ILM.

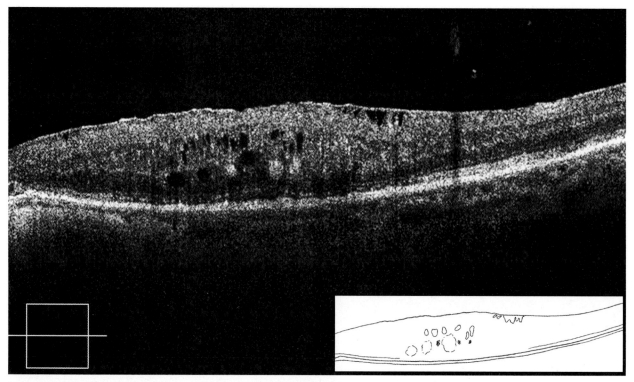

FIGURE 8. QUALITATIVE ANALYSIS – MORPHOLOGY – MACULAR PUCKER.
The ILM is thickened and irregular, with visible vitreoretinal traction and epiretinal membranes. The underlying retina is thickened by diffuse edema, with a few small pseudocysts mostly in the internal nuclear layer but also in the external nuclear layer.

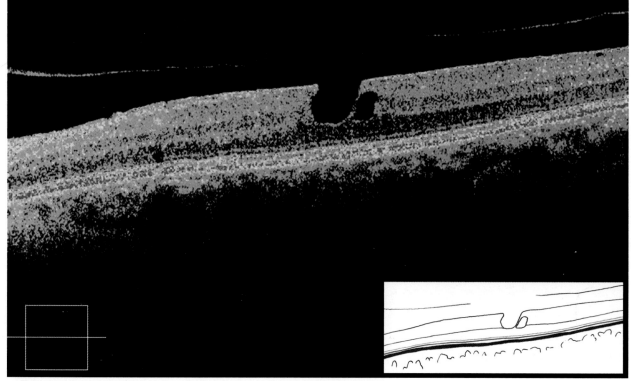

FIGURE 9. QUALITATIVE ANALYSIS – MORPHOLOGY – LAMELLAR HOLE.
A loss of internal layers of the retina and good preservation of the external layers can be observed here. The ELM and the IS/OS junction of the photoreceptors are visible.

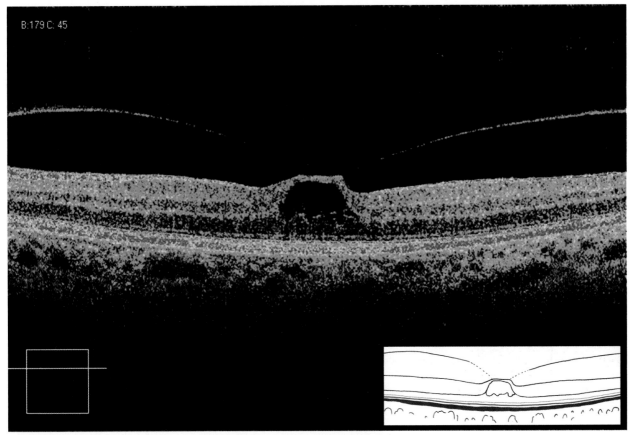

FIGURE 10. QUALITATIVE ANALYSIS—MORPHOLOGY – STAGE I MACULAR HOLE.
In this typical case, a large cystic structure in the internal layers of the retina is visible, while part of the normal retinal structure is preserved.

■ *Stage 4:* The hole is full-thickness, with loss of retinal substance, retinal edema on the margins, and detachment of the margins **(Figures 11, 12)**.

INTRARETINAL MORPHOLOGICAL ALTERATIONS

In this section, we discuss intraretinal fissures, where the retinal surface is not compromised. When the retinal surface is intact, macular pseudoholes can form a retinal fissure, called an impending hole, and then enlarge.

Posterior Morphological Alterations

These anomalies, especially serous or hemorrhagic detachments, are observed at the RPE level. Serous RPE detachments deform the posterior border of the retina and form an angle of more than 45° with Bruch's membrane and the choriocapillaris. Serous detachments of the neuroepithelium are less elevated and form angle of less than 45° with the RPE.

Retinal Pigment Epithelium

In cases of atrophy, the RPE deteriorates, revealing Bruch's membrane. The RPE can deteriorate irregularly, revealing one or more of the three normal layers.

In cases of neovascular membranes, we can observe dissociation and increased thickness of the RPE. Drusen are seen as irregular undulations, with slightly hyperreflective content **(Figure 13)**. Serous detachments, on the other hand, often have an optically blank or slightly vascularized appearance. It is then possible to observe Bruch's membrane as a thin, rectilinear line.

Retinal External Nuclear Layer

The external nuclear layer (ENL) gives information about the function of the photoreceptors. It can present as normal, or with the following:

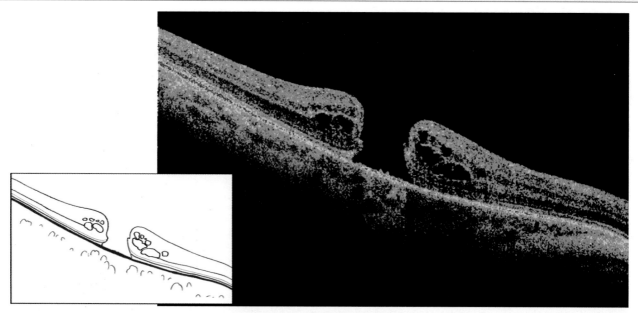

FIGURE 11. QUALITATIVE ANALYSIS – MORPHOLOGY – STAGE IV MACULAR HOLE.

The hole penetrates all layers, with only the RPE visible. Marked CME is thickening the margins of the hole, which are slightly detached from the RPE.

These pseudocysts are located in the internal and external nuclear layers. It is important to measure all components of the hole and its dimensions at different levels to decide if surgical intervention is necessary and to follow progression. The ILM and the IS/OS junction are normal in the surrounding retina and slightly detached at the margins of the hole. They disappear around the fovea with the rest of the retinal tissue. The rounded central hole, surrounded by a crown of regular pseudocystic cavities is visible in the frontal section.

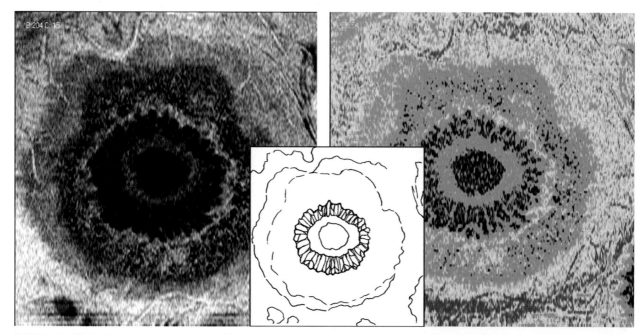

FIGURE 12. QUALITATIVE ANALYSIS – MORPHOLOGY – FRONTAL SECTION ADAPTED TO RPE CONTOUR – STAGE IV MACULAR HOLE.

This is a frontal image of the macular hole in Figure 11. The same scan is represented in gray scale and color scale. An oval hole at the center of the fovea is visible, surrounded by relatively regular cystic formations, elongated toward the center and inside the margins of the hole. The margins of the hole are thickened because they intersect the ILM and the IS/OS junction, which point toward one another.

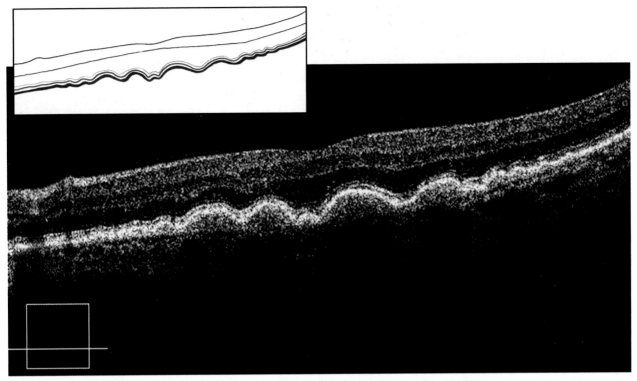

FIGURE 13. QUALITATIVE ANALYSIS – MORPHOLOGY – DEEP ANOMALOUS STRUCTURES – DRUSEN.
Undulations and a localized increase in thickness of the RPE/choriocapillaris corresponding to drusen can be seen. The ELM and the IS/OS junction are preserved, following the undulations of the RPE. A medium reflective substance fills the drusen. Bruch's membrane may be visible as a thin line.

- Increased foveal or localized thickness
- Diminished foveal or localilzed thickness
- Globally diminished or increased thickness
- Total absence of the ENL
- Presence of edema near the RPE layer
- Presence of exudates or other material at the RPE layer.

Any of these characteristics will give indications on the integrity of the photoreceptors, especially when compared with other indications. The junction of the internal and external segments of the photo-receptors (IS/OS junction) and the external segments

of the photoreceptors are also important **(Figure 14)**. The appearance can be linear; the junction can be deformed by folds and RPE detachments, or it can be thickened and altered, absent, or not visible.

External Limiting Membrane

The external limiting membrane (ELM) is normally more resilient than the IS/OS junction. It can be observed after the junction has disappeared. The ELM can be linear, broken, deformed by folds or RPE detachments, or altered in various ways. In some lesions, the ELM is absent.

TABLE 3: IS/OS JUNCTION POSSIBLE OCT MORPHOLOGIES
• Normal linear aspect
• Broken
• Deformed by folds or RPE detachments
• Thickened
• Absent

TABLE 4: EXTERNAL LIMITING MEMBRANE POSSIBLE OCT MORPHOLOGIES
• Normal linear aspect
• Broken
• Deformed by folds or RPE detachments
• Altered
• Absent

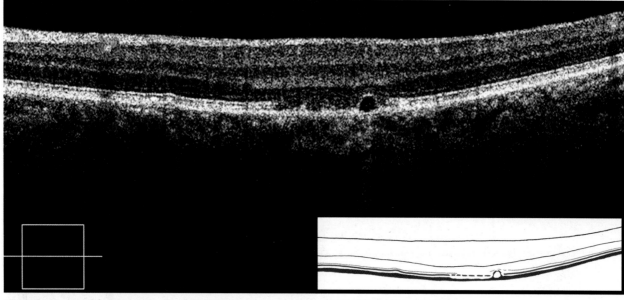

FIGURE 14. QUALITATIVE ANALYSIS – MORPHOLOGY – ALTERATIONS OF THE IS/OS JUNCTION.
A fundamental contribution of spectral domain OCT is that it allows us to visualize the various elements of the photoreceptors. We can see them well in this figure. The IS/OS junction normally presents as a hyperreflective line parallel to the RPE. Alterations of the photoreceptors appear as small breaks and irregularities. A slight thickening of the junction is associated with decreased thickness of the external nuclear layer. In this case, we also note the absence of the internal line of the RPE, which corresponds to the external segment of the photoreceptors. Do not confuse these irregularities with the shadows of the retinal blood vessels (visible in this image), which interrupt the IS/OS junction.

TABLE 5: EXTERNAL NUCLEAR LAYER POSSIBLE OCT MORPHOLOGIES
• Normal
• Increased foveal thickness
• Localized decreased thickness
• Thickness decreased globally
• Thickness increased in an organized manner
• Thickness increased globally
• Absence of the external nuclear layer
• Cystoid edema
• Exudates

TABLE 6: RETINAL PIGMENT EPITHELIUM POSSIBLE OCT MORPHOLOGIES
• Normal
• Increased thickness
• Decreased thickness
• Irregular thickness with one or two layers absent
• Anomalous appearance of layers
• Undulations (drusen)
• Detachments (serous RPE detachments)
• Three layers visible
• Layers not visible, fused
• Anomalous tissue in contact with the RPE: fibro-vascular tissue, active neovascular membranes, lipofuscin deposits
• RPE deformed by anomalous tissue

ANOMALOUS STRUCTURES

Because of increased scan density and higher resolution, SD-OCT provides improved evaluation of anomalous structures. The study of hyporeflective structures is easier, especially at the vitreous level and behind the RPE/choriocapillaris.

Pre-retinal and Epiretinal Membrane

The density, thickness, and location of preretinal and epiretinal membranes can be evaluated. The membrane may be adherent, fused with the internal limiting membrane (ILM), or fully or partially detached. Its reflectivity, however, is greater than the normal reflectivity of the RNFL.

Alterations of the profile or thickness of the membranes can indicate retinal traction. It can be separate from or adherent to the retina. It can cause

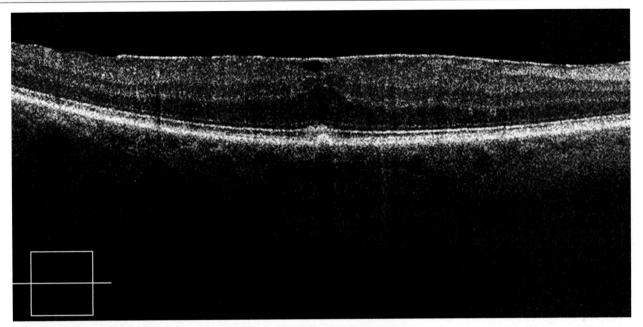

FIGURE 15. QUALITATIVE ANALYSIS – MORPHOLOGY – EPIRETINAL MEMBRANE.
This image shows partially detached epiretinal membrane combined in part with the RNFL. The foveal depression is absent. The retina is thickened, with diffuse edema.

wrinkles in the retinal surface. The preretinal or epiretinal membrane can be seen clearly as hyper-reflective because of thickening of the fibroglial elements.

If detached, the posterior hyaloid presents on OCT as a slightly reflective image, often broken and well-delineated, and adherent to the retina at some points **(Figure 15)**.

Macular Pucker

Retraction of the ILM is caused by a fibroglial proliferation, causing tangential traction. The force of this action creates retinal folds. Resultant changes occur to the courses of blood vessels, which appear elongated when parallel to the folds. Generally, retinal folds are transverse in the retina underlying the membrane and radial to that outside the area of traction.

Cotton Wool Spots

These hyperreflective formations are in contact with and often fused with the superficial RNFL. They are associated with ischemic lesions of the nerve fibers and are located at the periphery of the ischemic area.

Intraretinal Anomalous Structures

Hard exudates are localized in the posterior layers of the retina. They are formed from lipoproteins and can be isolated or part of the surrounding retina. They are found in the external plexiform layer at the boundary between the edematous area and the normal retina.

Posterior Anomalous Structures

Classic neovascular membranes are generally fusiform, nodular, rounded, and anterior to the RPE. If active, they are accompanied by edema or serous detachments of the neuroretina **(Figure 16; also see page 68, Figures 2A and 2B)**.

Occult neovascular membranes **(see page 69, Figure 3)** are more difficult to distinguish, presenting as a thickening of the RPE/choriocapillaris complex with a disassociated aspect. The active occult membranes are accompanied by diffuse or cystoid edema and localized serous detachments of the neuroretina.

Scars in advanced macular degeneration **(see page 70, Figure 7)** or diabetic fibrovascular membrane present as thickened areas of hyperreflective

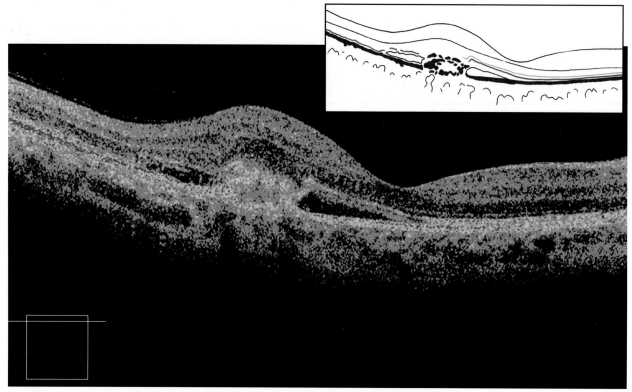

FIGURE 16. QUALITATIVE ANALYSIS – MORPHOLOGY – CLASSIC NEOVASCULAR MEMBRANE.
In this case of age-related macular degeneration, the neovascular membrane is elongated, fusiform, and located in front of the RPE. The lesions of the RPE and Bruch's membrane can be distinguished. Note the serous detachment of the neuroretina and the diffuse edema that surrounds it. In this case, pseudocystic cavities of edema do not appear. Edema and detachments of the neuroretina are always present with active nerve fiber membranes, whether they are classic or occult.

fibrovascular tissue. These scars distort the profile of the retina and can cause the normal elements of the retina to disappear.

3-D STUDY OF MORPHOLOGY

Analytical studies provided by the Cirrus™ HD-OCT software include 3-D imaging and frontal or coronal (*en face*) images, such as C-scan and RPE-fit **(Figure 17)**. These studies enable global evaluation of retinal changes.

We have only recently begun using the 3-D study of retinal pathology, but already we are improving our comprehension of certain diseases, such as cystoid macular edema (CME), pseudocysts within a full-thickness macular hole or a lamellar hole, serous detachments of the RPE or neuroepithelium, to name a few.

QUALITATIVE ANALYSIS: REFLECTIVITY

The study of reflectivity with SD-OCT does not precisely correspond to the same study done with time domain OCT, because we are better able to visualize structures with SD-OCT. One of the fundamental elements in OCT analysis is the ability to assess reflectivity. Reflectivity can be increased or decreased, or there can be a shadow zone. Collections of fluid are particularly easy to detect. For example, neovascular membranes examined with time domain OCT appear dense and homogeneous, while the same membranes examined with spectral domain OCT show dense zones and less reflective zones, with evident heterogeneity.

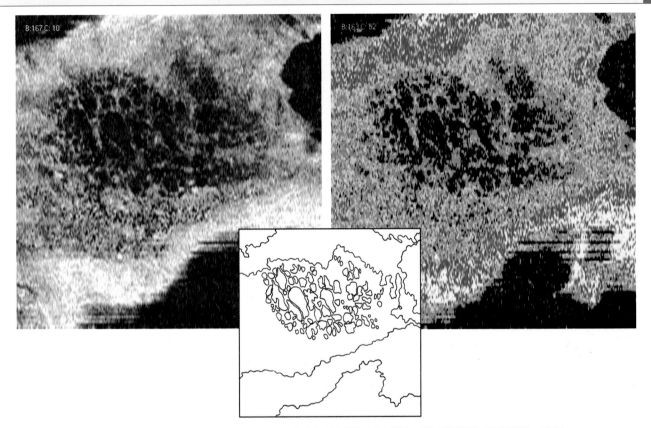

FIGURE 17. QUALITATIVE ANALYSIS – MORPHOLOGY – FRONTAL SECTION ADAPTED TO THE RPE CONTOUR – CME.
This is an *en face* view of diabetic retinopathy in a patient 12 years post diabetes diagnosis. The retina is thickened by diffuse and pseudocystic edema. Pseudocystic formations are developing in the periphery, especially at the external and internal nuclear layers. At the fovea, the cysts coalesced into oval cavities with vertical major axes, owing to the anatomical structure of the fovea. The pseudocysts vary in size; some are small and rounded, while others are irregular, formed by the merger of multiple pseudocysts.

HIGH REFLECTIVITY

The strength of the signal reflected from tissue depends on the following factors:

- The quantity of light when it arrives at a particular layer, having been partially absorbed by intervening tissues
- The quantity of light reflected
- The quantity of light reflected that reaches the detector after having been reabsorbed.

Horizontal anatomical structures, such as the nerve fibers and the plexiform layers, are more reflective than vertical structures.

Increased reflectivity may be superficial, intra-retinal or deep. Depending on its location, increased reflectivity may indicate the following:

Superficial

- Syndromes of the vitreoretinal interface, epiretinal or retinal fibrosis, macular pucker, pre-retinal or epiretinal membranes
- Superficial hemorrhage: dense, with a shadow effect of underlying structures; cotton wool spots are superficial with margins indistinct from the margins of areas of recent ischemia.

Intraretinal

- Lesions of the photoreceptors: in these cases, the IS/OS junction shows irregularity, interruptions and areas in which it is no longer visible. In cases of retinal atrophy, the ELM is more resistant, remaining visible longer.

TABLE 7: DETERMINANTS OF REFLECTIVITY ON SD-OCT
HIGHEST • Accumulation of pigment • Hypertrophy of the RPE • Choroidal nevus • Scar tissue **HIGH** • Nerve fiber (normal) • IS/OS junction (normal) • External segments of the photoreceptors • External limiting membrane • RPE/choriocapillaris complex (normal) • Hemorrhage • Neovascular membrane • Hard exudate **MEDIUM** • Plexiform layer (normal) • Retinal edema **LOW** • Nuclear layer (normal) • Collections of fluid: cavity, cyst, detachment • Shadow

TABLE 8: CAUSES OF HYPERREFLECTIVITY ON SD-OCT
SUPERFICIAL • Epiretinal or intraretinal fibrosis • Cotton wool spots **INTRARETINAL** • Inflammatory infiltrate • Hemorrhage • Hard exudates • Intraretinal neovascularization **DEEP** • Accumulation of lipofuscin • Hyperplasia of the RPE • Atrophy of the RPE with retrodiffusion • Classic or occult neovascular membranes

- Retinal serous detachments: as in serous chorioretinitis, the external segment of the photoreceptors, which can be thickened, irregular or have increased reflectivity, presents granulations or flaking of the internal face of the detachment in the detached area.
- Hemorrhage: dense, with a shadow effect.
- Hard exudate: nodular, hyperreflective zones composed of lipoproteins at the boundary between the healthy retina and the edematous retina. They are generally located in deep layers.

Deep

- Drusen cause an undulation or localized increase in thickness of the RPE/choriocapillaris complex.
- Pre- and retroepithelial neovascular membranes that merge with the RPE complex: Bruch's membrane and choriocapillaris show increased reflectivity under a thin retina.
- Scars from choroiditis, traumatic lesions, retinal fibrosis, disciform degeneration. Recent laser impacts are seen as vertical, hyperreflective stripes leading from the RNFL to the RPE. Because of hyperpigmentation, those in the choroid appear as increased reflectivity in the RPE/choriocapillaris complex, and cause a shadow zone **(Figure 18)**. Increased retrodiffusion of light may indicate atrophy of the retina and the RPE.

LOW REFLECTIVITY

Decreased reflectivity may be caused by less reflective tissue, such as atrophied RPE with less pigment **(Figure 19)**. Collections of fluid may by seen as cysts or hemorrhagic detachment of the neuroretina or RPE **(Figure 20 and 21)**.

Areas of low reflectivity may be minimal or extensive. They take on an important role in 3-D studies and frontal scans.

- *Low intraretinal reflectivity.* Edema, CME, cyst, microcyst, impending hole.
- *Low subintraretinal reflectivity.* Serous detachment of the neuroretina. The detachment forms an acute angle with the RPE.

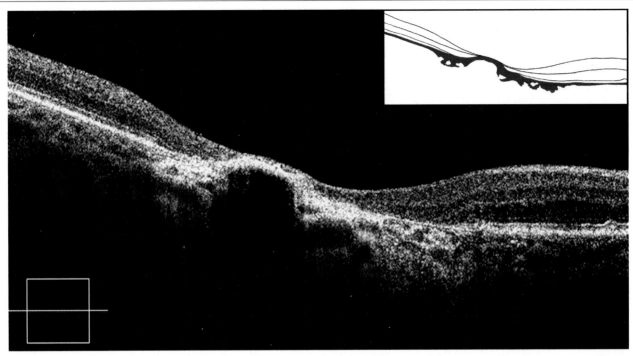

FIGURE 18. QUALITATIVE ANALYSIS – REFLECTIVITY – HYPERPIGMENTATION FROM CHORIORETINAL SCARRING AND FIBROSIS.
A densely pigmented scar and marked thinning of the adjacent retina is observed. This pigmentation casts a dense shadow on the posterior layers.

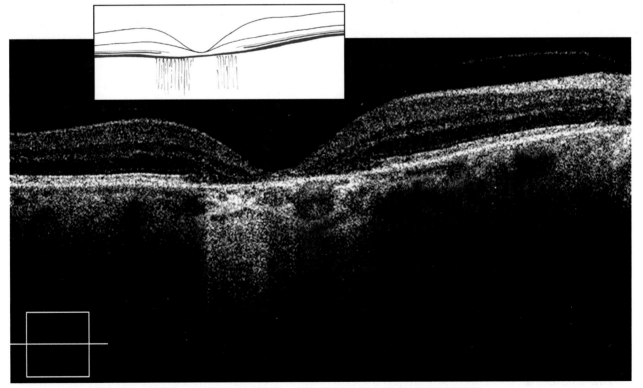

FIGURE 19. QUALITATIVE ANALYSIS – LOW REFLECTIVITY – RETRODIFFUSION FROM RPE ATROPHY.
Atrophy of the retina and the RPE is characterized by a marked decrease in retinal thickness. The hyporeflective, atrophied RPE and the reduced thickness of the retina allow more light to penetrate the choroid. Less light is absorbed crossing the retina, and the light reflected is also absorbed less as it returns. At the margins of the atrophied zone, the thickness of the external nuclear layer is normal, and the ELM and the IS/OS junction can be seen.

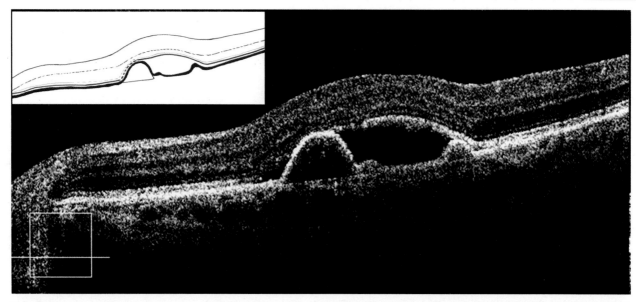

FIGURE 20. QUALITATIVE ANALYSIS – REFLECTIVITY – RPE DETACHMENT WITH DETACHED NEUROEPITHELIUM IN SEROUS CHORIORETINOPATHY.

In this case, the contents of the RPE detachment are clear. The detachment forms an obtuse angle with a portion of the RPE still attached. Bruch's membrane is visible as a thin line, detached from the RPE, having remained horizontal. In this serous RPE detachment, the thickness of the boundary is regular and the internal boundaries are smooth. The RPE detachment is associated with a small detachment of the neuroepithelium.

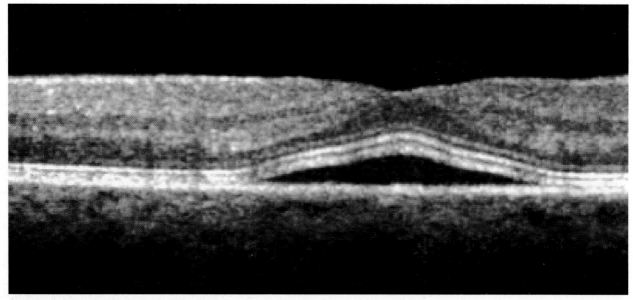

FIGURE 21. DETACHED NEUROEPITHELIUM.

This image shows a detachment of the neuroepithelium in a case of central serous chorioretinopathy. The margins of the detachment form an acute angle with the RPE, and the ILM follows the detachment. The line of the IS/OS junction follows the changes from the detachment. The RPE/choriocapillaris complex, which spectral domain OCT sees as two reflective lines separated by a minimal hyporeflective line, shows a fissure. The superior line is separated from the RPE and forms the inferior boundary of the serous detachment. This is formed by the external segment of the photoreceptors. In cases of prolonged detachment, the segments of the photoreceptors, which form the anterior boundary of the detachment, become altered and indistinct, indicating alterations of the photoreceptors.

- *Low reflectivity under the RPE.* Serous detachments of the RPE that has separated from Bruch's membrane. The fluid from the choriocapillaris accumulates in the subepithelial space, creating an obtuse angle with the underlying layers.

Serous detachments can be idiopathic, associated with acute or chronic central serous chorioretinopathy or secondary to serous or hemorrhagic disciform degeneration. Rarer causes may include myopia, angioid streaks, choroiditis, and choroidal neoformations. Often, they are associated with the presence of a neovascular membrane. The area of the detachment or the cystic space can be optically blank in cases of serous detachment or more reflective in cases of inflammatory exudations or senile degeneration.

- *Hemorrhagic.* The detachment shows areas that are not optically blank; they may be shadowed by highly reflective areas.
- *Diminution of the pigment in the atrophized area of the pigment epithelium.*

SHADOW ZONES

Dense, reflective tissue may create a shadow on posterior elements. The highly sensitive spectral domain instruments lend far more contrast to the shadow zone determined by the retinal blood vessels and intraretinal reflective formations. At the IS/OS junction and the ILM, the shadow of the retinal blood vessels obscures these structures and simulates lesions of the photoreceptors **(Figure 22)**.

The structures of the retina can be occluded at various levels: preretinal, intraretinal, and posterior. We have noted the following with regard to shadows apparent in spectral domain OCT studies.

Anterior Level

The normal retinal blood vessels are difficult to distinguish, but they cast a cone of shadow that allows us to find them. Superficial or profound hemorrhage causes a cone of shadow, as do cotton wool exudates.

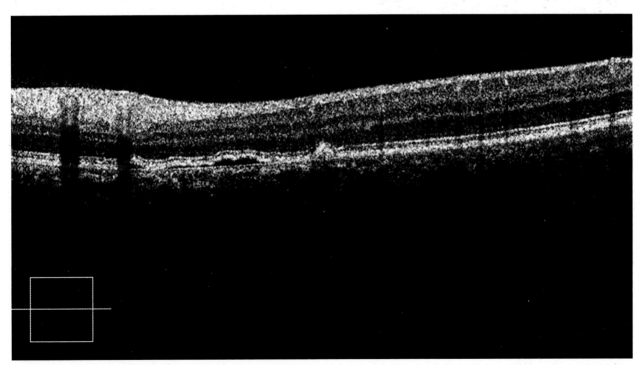

FIGURE 22. SHADOW OF NORMAL RETINAL BLOOD VESSELS.
In spectral domain OCT scans, the normal retinal blood vessels, which are difficult to observe in the RNFL, form vertical shadows that interrupt the underlying structures. It is important to recognize these to avoid confusing the interruptions of the ILM and the IS/OS junction with true alterations of the photoreceptors. Spectral domain OCT shows the blood vessel itself or its contents if the vessel is large.

Posterior Level

Hard lipid exudates in the deep retinal layers cast dense shadows. Pigmented areas can form a screen with an inclined shadow. Hyperplasia and hypertrophy of the RPE are seen as dense shadows.

Neovascularization of the choroid is detected by an increase in reflectivity in the RPE/Bruch's membrane complex and a slight increase in the thickness of this layer, with a shadow cast on the posterior layers.

A dense, pigmented scar casts a shadow. A markedly hyperreflective subretinal neovascular membrane, if thick, also casts a shadow.

QUANTITATIVE ANALYSIS

Quantification is an important aspect of an analytic examination. It allows comparison of numerical data in the natural course of a disease or its response to therapy. With certain software, we can quantify the thickness of the retina or retinal elements (for example, the RNFL in glaucoma), as well as the volume of the retina. Spectral domain OCT provides better definition and contrast between the retinal layers, allowing precise study and measurement of various layers.

In lesions of the internal retina due to occlusions of the retinal venules or arterioles, there are marked variations of the nerve fibers, the ganglion layer, the internal plexiform layer, and the internal nuclear layer. In venous occlusions and recent arterial occlusions, there is an increase in thickness. In arterial occlusions, after a few weeks, a marked reduction in internal retinal thickness appears. The external nuclear layer is the most important layer of the external retina to evaluate because you can detect damage to the photoreceptors.

Time domain OCT automatically measures retinal thickness, showing the distance between the vitreoretinal interface and the anterior surface of the pigment epithelium, which varies from 275 to 200 microns. The foveal depression varies from 190 to 170 microns. At the fovea, the average thickness is approximately 170 to 190 microns; and the peripheral

TABLE 9: CAUSES FOR SHADOWING EFFECT ON SD-OCT
ANTERIOR
• Hemorrhage
• Exudates
• Retinal blood vessels (normal)
POSTERIOR
• Neovascular membranes
• RPE thickening
• Accumulation of pigment
• Choroidal neovascularization
• Retinal scar

retina is 240 microns. The retinal fibers are thicker in the interpapillomacular area. The nerve fibers form a slightly thickened arc of about 500 microns within the fovea, normally reaching 270 microns. The thickness is measured on single scans and over the retinal map. The normative database software enables us to compare variations to the normal eye.

Spectral domain OCT gives higher values for retinal thickness because it identifies the RPE more precisely than time domain OCT, which confuses it with the IS/OS junction.

RETINAL THICKNESS VARIATIONS

With the retinal map, we can immediately visualize areas of increased or decreased thickness. With Cirrus™ HD-OCT, we can also evaluate the volume of the retina, enabling us to follow the progression of edema or atrophy more precisely **(Figures 23, 24)**.

Increased thickness may be observed in the following:

■ **Retinal edema.** This is the most frequent cause of retinal thickening. Our improved ability to study and evaluate the various forms of retinal edema constitutes one of the major advances of OCT. The three stages of retinal edema are: simple edema, cystoid macular edema (CME), and chronic edema with serous detachment of the retina. The presence of collected liquid in the retinal layers or in front of the RPE indicates increased retinal thickness.

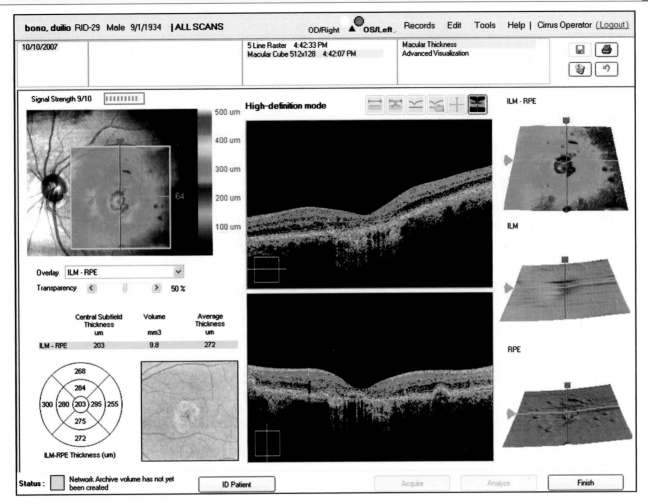

FIGURE 23. RETINAL ATROPHY.
The marked decrease in retinal thickness is shown numerically and by conventional colors. The software also calculates the volume and average thickness of the retina. At the side, we can see the 3-D view of the retinal thickness, the ILM, which appears altered, and the RPE, which is altered.

- **Vitreoretinal traction.** This is caused when the ERM from diabetic retinopathy or interface syndromes pulls the superficial layers of the retina, with deformations in the profile and secondary edema.

Decreased thickness may be observed in the following:

- **Atrophic degeneration.** At the posterior pole, we can see a marked decrease in retinal thickness to 150 or even 100 microns. We also can see areas of RPE atrophy, which are thinner and less reflective owing to loss of pigment. The hyporeflective RPE allows increased penetration of light into the choroid. The reflectivity is increased because light absorption is reduced at the retina and the RPE.

- **Laser scars, fibrous scars.** Scars consequent to laser treatment, chorioretinitis or trauma indicate atrophy of the retina, with thickening of the pigment epithelium/choriocapillaris complex.

VARIATIONS IN THICKNESS OF RETINAL LAYERS

Various pathologies cause the retina to become thicker or thinner in certain areas and in well-defined layers. The images and the retinal maps generated by OCT enable us to precisely locate and track disease progression.

Morphological alterations may involve the entire retina or the retinal surface, with changes to the foveal and extrafoveal retinal profile.

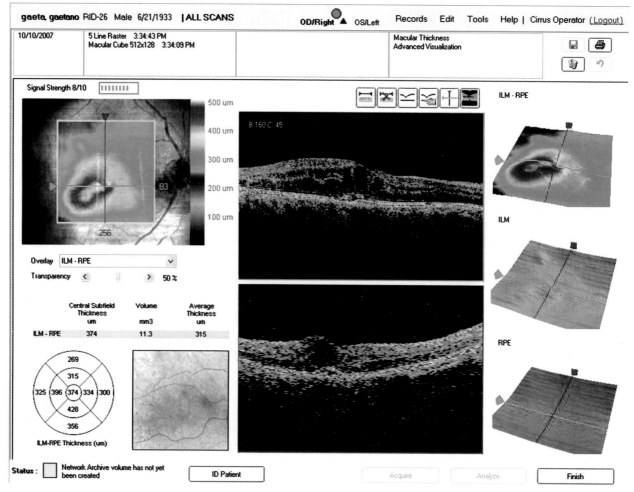

FIGURE 24. EDEMA.
Note the marked increase in retinal thickness, shown numerically and by conventional colors. The software also calculates the volume and average thickness of the retina. The 3-D view of the retinal thickness is shown with an altered ILM and a normal RPE.

In glaucoma, study of RNFL thickness variations is important when examined on circular chorioretinal scans of the papilla.

MACULAR RETINAL MAP: TIME DOMAIN VS. SPECTRAL DOMAIN

A retinal map uses color coding to describe the thickness of the posterior pole as follows:

- White: greater than 450 micron
- Red: 350 to 450 microns
- Orange: 320 to 350
- Yellow: 270 to 320 microns
- Green: 170 to 250 microns
- Blue: less than 170 microns.

Time Domain OCT

The time domain retinal map is created from six consecutive OCT tomograms, following a star-like pattern that intersects at the fovea. Thickness measurements are taken at 100 points in each tomogram, with a total of 600 points, six of which coincide at the foveola. Thus, the measurements are more precise in the center of the map than in the periphery. The software calculates average thicknesses.

The results are shown in two modes. A quantitative interpretation includes a central subfield with a diameter of 500 microns and two concentric rings subdivided into four quadrants each. The average thickness is reported in each defined area.

A topographical map in false colors also is created. The normal retinal map appears green (200-250 microns) with a blue fovea (170 microns). The instrument calculates the estimated thickness in each slice of the retina between tomograms.

Spectral Domain OCT

Spectral domain retinal maps incorporate several important advances. For example, spectral domain OCT acquires 200 to 512 B-scans from top to bottom in rapid succession. The software then constructs a retinal map by aligning the B-scans. The high acquisition speed and finer scan grid allow a high degree of accuracy and more detailed maps.

The calculation of the average thickness with grids and quadrants is improved by new software that corrects for artifacts, such as those created by media opacity or markedly altered macular morphology **(Figures 23, 24)**.

With this technology, we can determine RNFL thickness and the profile of each scan, compare the average RNFL thickness to a normal age-matched population, and create a map of the RNFL.

RETINAL VOLUME

In addition to creating a retinal thickness map, the spectral domain OCT software calculates the retinal volume for each map. This is important for following the progression of edema or a serous detachment, either the natural history or after laser or surgical intervention. This technology is indispensable for studying the effects of pharmacological intervention.

TABLE 10: QUANTITATIVE ANALYTICAL STUDY OF THE RETINA
RETINAL THICKNESS • Increased • Decreased • Variations in thickness of a layer (e.g., nerve fibers) • Retinal map • Volume

DATA SYNTHESIS

Synthesis is the most important aspect of the diagnostic assessment, because only a complete analysis of all data will produce a precise, well-founded diagnosis.

In the overall evaluation, the clinician also must use data that is not directly associated with OCT. Factor such as the patient's age, current health status, general and ocular health history, visual acuity, ocular status via clinical examination, and additional studies, such as fluorescein angiography and indocyanine green angiography, are important.

It is essential to study angiograms at all time sequences and to compare them with the analyzed elements of hyper- and hyporeflectivity, and morphological factors, retinal thickness, the retinal map, and volumetry. It is also important to anatomically locate the hypo- and hyperreflective structures. Data on choroidal or retinal pathology may be shown that was not detected on a fundus photo or isolated scan. In certain cases, an anomalous ocular fundus may appear normal on OCT or vice versa. Combining all of these elements will lead to a true understanding and evaluation of OCT studies.

It is also important to study the three-dimensional views provided by the 3-D map, C-scan and RPE-fit images. When these seemingly disparate elements are analyzed together, they take on new significance and allow the global consideration of the ocular disease.

SUMMARY

Optical coherence tomography has enabled us to expand our knowledge of ocular disease by showing us pathology that was previously not well known. This technology has helped improve our understanding of the structure and pathophysiology of pseudoholes and macular holes, retinal traction, macular edema, serous detachments of the retina and RPE, and choroidal neovascularization and its evolution after therapy. In addition, it has modified our understanding of retinal disease and its progression, and changed the indications for vitreoretinal surgery.

Spectral domain OCT has helped us improve our knowledge of congenital retinoschisis, central serous retinopathies, the progression of neovascular membranes, and the presentation and progression of macular dystrophy and atrophic degeneration.

In addition, quantitative OCT is important for evaluating the efficacy of photodynamic therapy, classic laser therapy, and transpupillary thermotherapy.

We believe one of the most important applications for OCT is the evaluation of new therapies, such as intravitreal and retrobulbar antiangiogenics, and intravitreal therapeutic implants, and the effects of therapy in general on ocular pathology. In these cases, it helps us to decide if and when we should repeat therapy, according to the degree of retinal edema, fibrosis, or atrophy.

TABLE 11: SD-OCT PROVIDES IMPROVED CLINICAL UTILITY IN THE STUDY OF THE FOLLOWING

- Alterations of the photoreceptors
- External limiting membrane
- Retinal pigment epithelium
- Bruch's membrane
- Retinal map
- Macular degeneration
- Macular retinoschisis
- Acute and chronic retinal epitheliopathy
- Traumatic epitheliopathy
- Branch vein occlusion
- Arterial occlusion
- Solar retinopathy
- Acute retinitis
- White dot syndromes

- Vitreous and epiretinal membrane
- Vitreous opacity
- Vitreoretinal interface
- Cystoid macular edema
- Epiretinal membrane
- Vitreoretinal traction
- Lamellar holes and holes at all thicknesses
- Retinal pigment epithelium atrophy
- Hyaloidal interface abnormalities
- Diffuse edema
- Syndromes of the vitreoretinal interface
- Macular pucker
- Diabetic retinopathy

TABLE 12: DATA SYNTHESIS FOR DIAGNOSIS

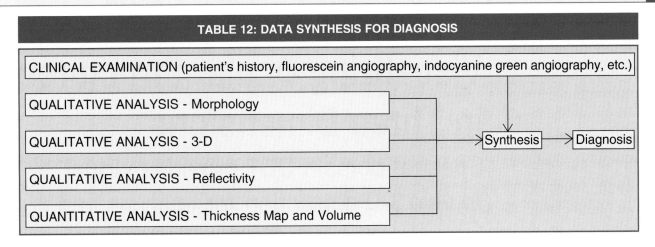

TABLE 13: QUALITATIVE ANALYTICAL STUDY HYPOREFLECTIVITY

Optically Blank Spaces
- Cysts, microcysts, cavities
- Intraretinal edema
- Exudative detachments of the neuroepithelium
- Cystoid macular edema
- RPE detachments
- RPE hypopigmentation

TABLE 14: QUALITATIVE ANALYTICAL STUDY BOUNDARIES OF RPE DETACHMENTS

- Regular, rounded
- Single or multiple
- Irregular
- Smooth
- Bumpy

Chapter 4

Visualizing Ocular Structures in Three Dimensions

Spectral domain OCT provides virtual *in vivo* 3-D dissection for analysis and interpretation of retinal pathology.

A new and important aspect of spectral domain optical coherence tomography (SD-OCT) is its ability to produce three-dimensional (3-D) and frontal or coronal (*en face*) images adapted to the scleral curvature. With these images, global evaluation of abnormalities is simpler than with two-dimensional B-scan studies.

Using SD-OCT, we can choose from four views: a 3-D image, a 2-D cross section, a C-scan (i.e., flat *en face* sections of the retina), or the RPE-fit display, which compares a patient's retinal pigment epithelium (RPE) to a normal parabolic RPE, enabling us to detect variations from normal.

3-D STUDIES

To acquire a 3-D study of a macular cube, the instrument performs multiple scans at high resolution. Serial acquisition of B-scans for the retinal map provides a true representation of tissue for measurement and cross-sectional analysis. Three-dimensional images of the principal structures on which topographical calculation is based are displayed on screen. The study shows a cross section of retinal tissue, with the image of the fundus aligned below it **(Figures 1A-1E).**

It takes 1.6 seconds to acquire 200 horizontal scans (B-scans) with 200 scan lines each on the Y axis (A-scans). Average foveal thickness is 160 to 180 microns, so the theoretical resolution of the A-scan analysis is less than 4 microns.

The 3-D images can be displayed in different analysis formats. The most widely used is the Macular Thickness Analysis. The graphic on the right side of the macular map in the Macular Thickness Analysis shows the distance between the internal limiting membrane (ILM) and the RPE, using a cold/warm color scale to differentiate the measure of thickness. Below that are the segmented layers of the ILM (pale blue) and the RPE/choriocapillaris complex (brown or cream) **(see page 47, Figure 2).**

These images can be studied independently or in combination with the 3-D color map of the retina. A precise point of the B-scan where the lesion is located can be selected and rotated for display.

These images are useful for qualitative study of the pathology of the vitreoretinal interface, macular degeneration, and significant lesions, such as RPE atrophy, as they appear in the B-scan. They also have great didactic value for explaining how lesions present.

C-SCAN BY OCT

In the Advanced Visualization Analysis, it is possible to study the coronal or C-scans. These images show clinically important views, allowing us to plot the axial images (B-scans) over areas not routinely explored.

C-SCAN (*EN FACE*) BY SPECTRAL DOMAIN OCT

Spectral domain OCT technology can calculate and reconstruct C-scans from the acquired macular cube. The starting point is the acquisition of a macular cube image, usually with the 512 × 128 protocol. An advanced calculation function aligns and extracts the coronal planes from the cube.

The analysis of a classic (planar) C-scan operates directly on a reference B-scan moving along a plane horizontal to the tissue, displaying the corresponding C-scan on a different area of the monitor **(Figures 1E and 4).**

RPE-FIT FUNCTION CIRRUS™ HD-OCT

The RPE-fit function of the Cirrus™ HD-OCT is an interesting and important innovation to advance our understanding of ocular pathology. It provides an improved C-scan adapted to the retinal curvature. With it, we can obtain *en face* images that follow the curvature of the posterior pole **(Figures 3, 5, 6)**.

The RPE-fit software identifies the RPE/choriocapillaris complex and displays it as a curved 3-D section plane. The RPE-fit technology is adapted to the concavity of the RPE/choriocapillaris. The transverse sections follow the shape of the globe, so that an RPE-fit layer is the virtual representation of an ideally parabolic RPE. This parabolic curve is normal for the eye studied and is a function of the complex curvature of the globe.

To obtain a more precise image, we can select the thickness of a section from 2 to 20 microns, depending on our needs for clinical study. Thin sections are called slices; thicker sections are called slabs.

EN FACE FUNCTION RTVUE 100 SD-OCT

It provides scans adapted to the cup-shaped curvature of the posterior pole. The images can be selected on the retinal surface, inside the retina or in the choroid and are similar to the ones we described.

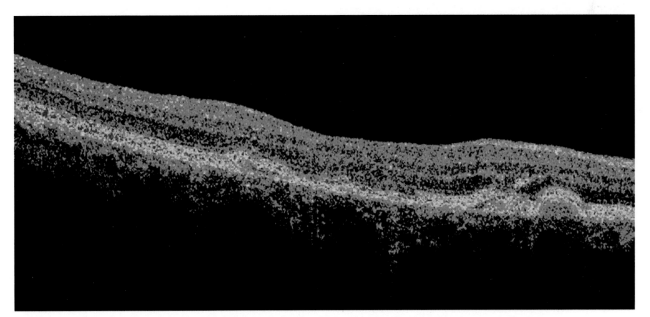

FIGURE 1A. COLOR B-SCAN OF AN EYE AFFECTED BY INCIPIENT AMD, NUMEROUS DRUSEN AND RPE DETACHMENTS.
The RPE thickness is slightly irregular with undulations formed by the drusen. The IS/OS junction is slightly irregular and altered at several points. The external limiting membrane is slightly altered, as is the thickness of the external nuclear layer. The drusen are slightly reflective. At some points where the RPE is detached, Bruch's membrane can be seen. In Figures 1B-1E, a 3-D cube of tissue relative to this scan is shown.

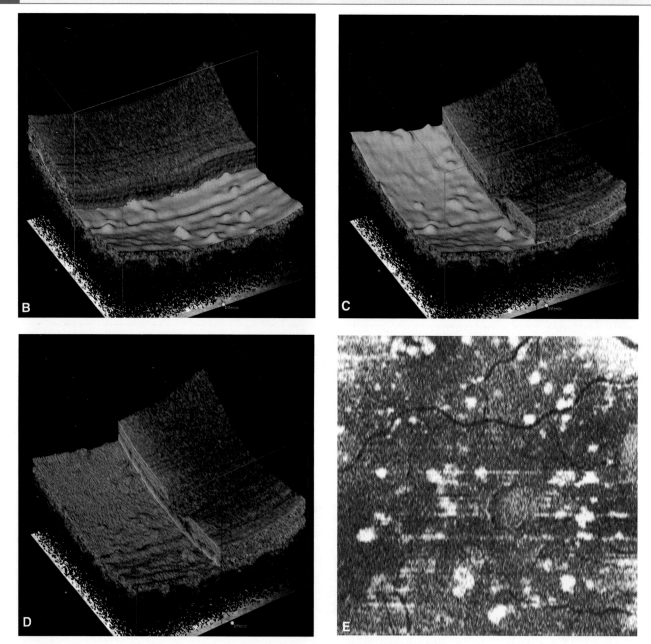

FIGURES 1B-E. 3-D STUDY OF A RETINAL CUBE RELATIVE TO AMD WITH NUMEROUS DRUSEN.

Figures 1B and 1C: These images are rotated to show different sides of the cube. Slices relative to the RPE elaborated by the software have been integrated with the cube. Integrations of other slices are also possible.

Figure 1D: The 3-D cube has been sectioned to remove part of the retina. The cube can be sectioned along the X-Y-Z axes. The color and transparency can be adjusted for better visualization of the deep and superficial layers.

Figure 1E: This graphic represents a frontal (transverse) C-scan section grazing the RPE, which sections the drusen along the epithelial slice.

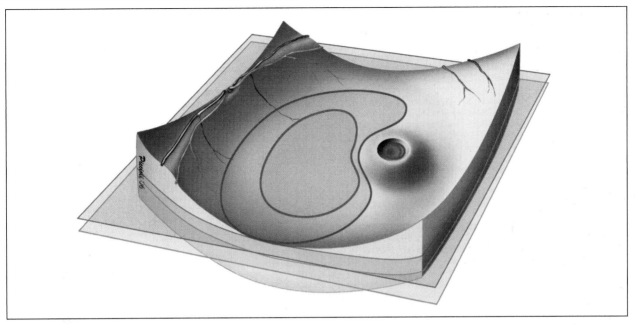

FIGURE 2. C-SCANS. 3-D VIEW OF THE OCULAR FUNDUS.
The posterior pole is shaped like a bowl, and the foveal area is shaped like a volcano. The C-scans are flat, sectioning the curvature of the posterior pole and showing a bean-shaped depression at the posterior pole and a rounded area near the fovea.

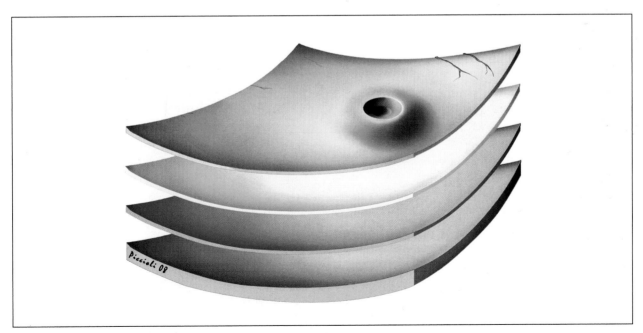

FIGURE 3. TRANSVERSE SECTIONS ADAPTED TO THE CURVATURE OF THE FUNDUS.
The retina is shown frontally, sectioned by scans following the average curvature of the posterior pole of the eye (RPEfit). We can see the posterior retina and three slices adapted to the concavity of the RPE/choriocapillaris. Thus, we can see transverse scans (slices or slabs) that are not flat, but follow the curved shape of the eye.

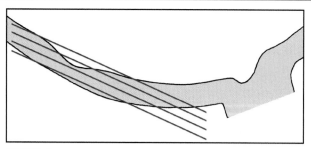

FIGURE 4.
Cross section of posterior pole and optic nerve, sectioned by four planes crossing the fovea.

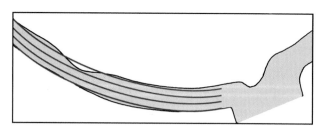

FIGURE 5.
Cross section of posterior pole and optic nerve, sectioned by four concave slices adapted to the average curvature of the RPE.

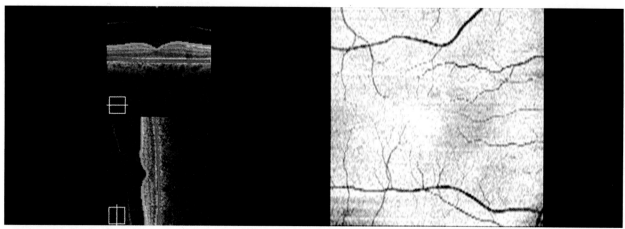

FIGURE 6. NORMAL RPE-fit.
Cirrus™ HD-OCT software uses the vitreoretinal interface as an internal marker and successively calculates the average curvature of the external marker. In this mode, an ideal concave surface is created, which slices and shows all retinal layers. The thickness of the slice can be adjusted to eliminate small artifacts, which can reduce sensitivity.

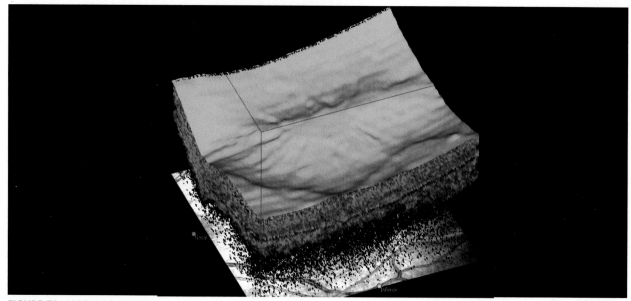

FIGURE 7A. MACULAR PUCKER.
The 3-D cube obtained using the Cirrus™ HD-OCT software shows the ILM. It is assumed that under a superficial membrane, there are striae radiating out from the center. The retraction of the ILM causes vitreoretinal traction toward the center, with formation of radial retinal folds.

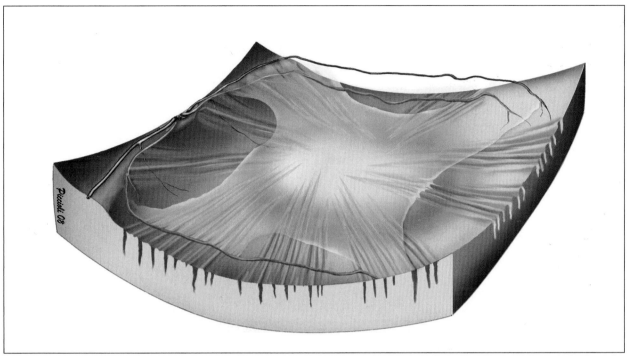

FIGURE 7B.
This illustration shows the ILM covering the posterior pole, the vitreoretinal adherence and the radial retinal folds.

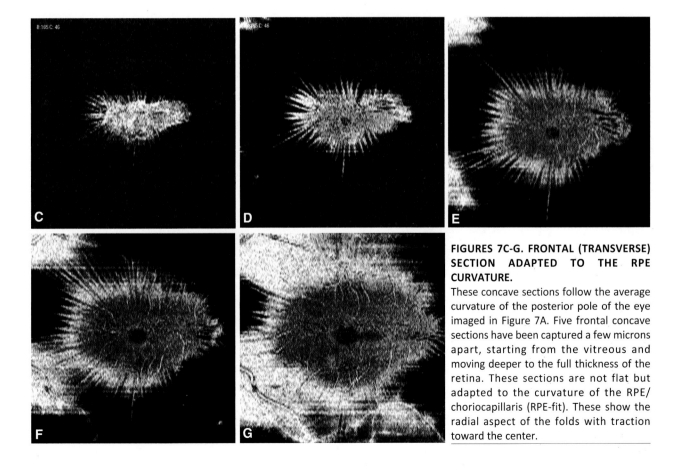

FIGURES 7C-G. FRONTAL (TRANSVERSE) SECTION ADAPTED TO THE RPE CURVATURE.

These concave sections follow the average curvature of the posterior pole of the eye imaged in Figure 7A. Five frontal concave sections have been captured a few microns apart, starting from the vitreous and moving deeper to the full thickness of the retina. These sections are not flat but adapted to the curvature of the RPE/choriocapillaris (RPE-fit). These show the radial aspect of the folds with traction toward the center.

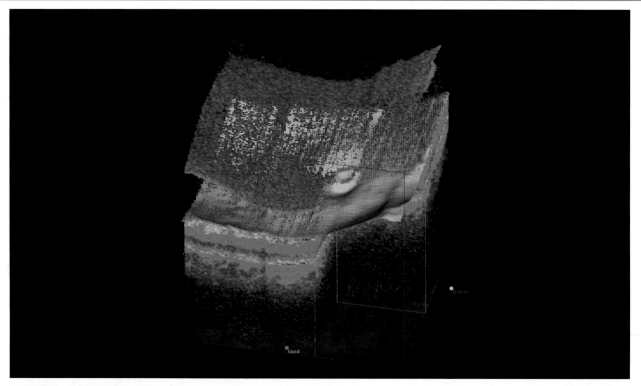

FIGURE 8A. ANTEROPOSTERIOR VITREORETINAL TRACTION – 3-D CUBE.
This cube has been sectioned to show the vitreous with vitreoretinal traction and the superficial film of the ILM. A part of the deep retina has been removed.

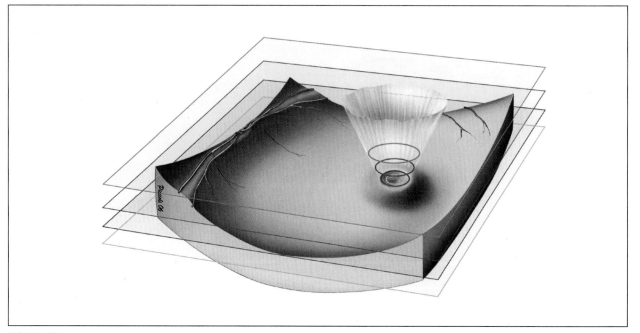

FIGURE 8B.
This illustration shows the posterior vitreous creating traction on the retina and the vitreoretinal adherences. Three frontal (transverse) sections have been designated, sectioning the vitreous and retina at various levels, showing the rings formed by the vitreal traction. The rings become progressively smaller as they approach the fovea.

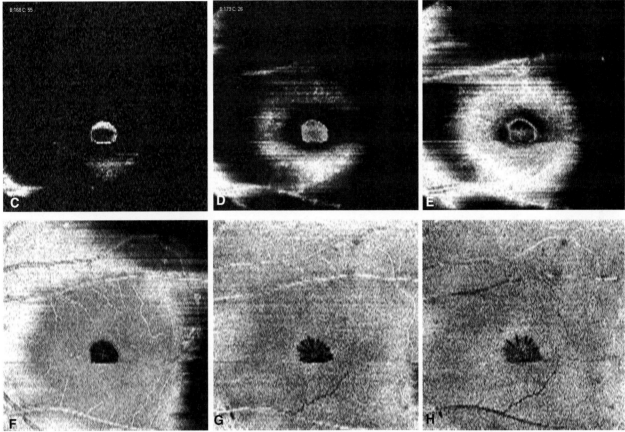

FIGURES 8C-H. ANTEROPOSTERIOR VITREORETINAL TRACTION – FRONTAL SECTIONS ADAPTED TO THE RPE CURVATURE.
These images correspond to the eye in Figure 8A. These six frontal sections are adapted to the curvature of the RPE/choriocapillaris (RPE-fit). They begin in the vitreous and move toward the choroid. The ring formed by the vitreal traction, the direct traction on the retina, and the hole forming deeper into the retina are shown. In the deepest layer, small radial cavities formed by the vitreal traction on the retinal tissue are shown.

Increasing the thickness of the RPE-fit section reduces the sensitivity of the technique but allows the study of deviations over a larger area. This mode provides an optimal display of the choroid. By changing the thickness of the section, we can display the medium and large blood vessels of the choroid with precision **(Figures 7C-H, 8C-H, 9B-E)**.

READING NORMAL C-SCAN CROSS-SECTIONS

One of the challenges in interpreting a C-scan is that it is a flat image of a concave structure. In addition, the thickness of the retina is not consistent, particularly near the foveal depression. The normal retinal surface has an irregularly undulating profile over the entire posterior pole, not only at the foveal depression. Thus, a horizontal surface scan can easily involve the layers of the nerve fibers and the foveal depression **(Figure 4)**.

With the Cirrus™ HD-OCT, we can study a pathologic lesion on a plane parallel to the RPE and observe the histological peculiarities relative to the disease in question. In a normal C-scan, the structures are often obliquely sectioned. The variations in tilt of the retina in relation to the coronal plane contribute to alterations in image orientation. This modality is extremely sensitive to small inclination of the eye, which can cause marked variations in the images.

CONCAVITY OF THE POSTERIOR POLE

As the flat C-scan moves deeper during a coronal examination, we first see the superficial retinal layers in the periphery, then the foveal depression, which

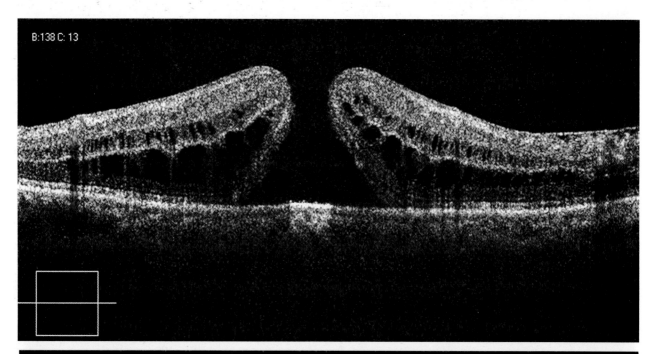

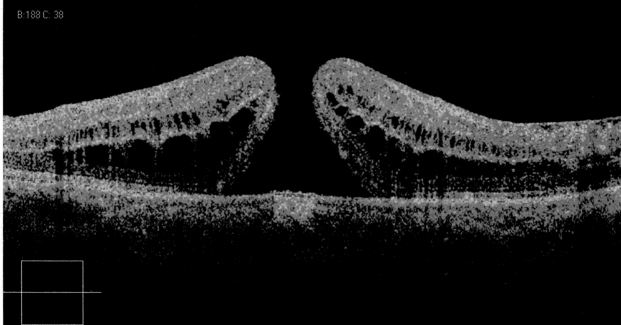

FIGURE 9A. B-SCAN OF STAGE IV MACULAR HOLE.

In this cross-section of a full-thickness macular hole, we can see the ILM and the IS/OS junction at the bottom. The diameter of the hole is smaller toward the vitreous, and it widens as it extends toward the RPE, giving it the classic anvil form. Small cysts occupy the internal and external nuclear layer. The external cystic formations are long and irregular. The cystic formations at the internal nuclear layer are small and irregular.

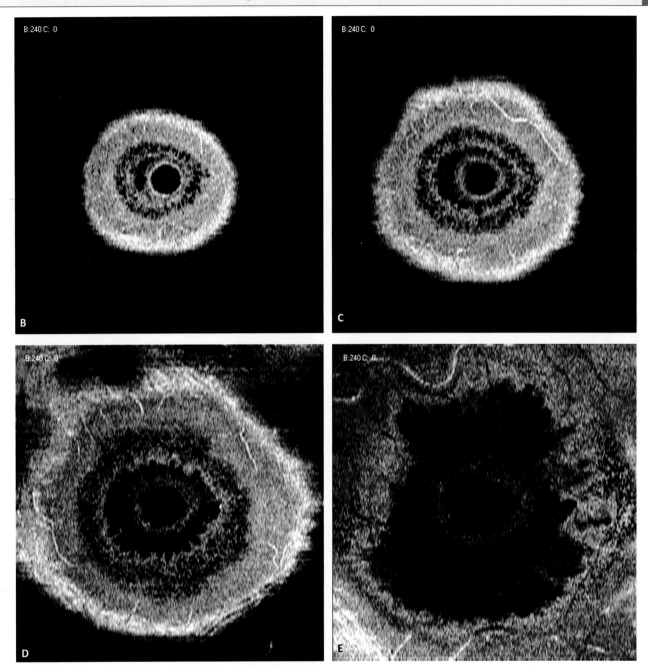

FIGURES 9B-E. MACULAR HOLE – FRONTAL SECTIONS ADAPTED TO THE RPE CURVATURE.

These images correspond to the eye in Figure 9A. They show four levels of the macular hole, starting in the vitreous and moving toward the choroid.

Figure 9B is a superficial view, showing the regular, rounded macular hole, surrounded by a ring of cystoid edema and a half-ring concentric with the hole.

Figure 9C, a deeper section, shows the central hole with thicker boundaries surrounded by two rings of cystoid edema cells. These rings are independent of one another with no contact between the cells of the two rings.

At an even deeper level (Figure 9D), the central hole is still visible with thick boundaries and two rings of edematous cells. The section appears as a hyperreflective surface without edematous lesions.

The last section (Figure 9E) is close to the RPE level. The macular hole is wider here than in the superficial sections. A central ring of cystoid edema can be seen surrounding the hole, and the cells of the cystoid edema clearly are in contact with one another. The cells have a radial aspect, starting from the center. The central hole has a rounded, thick boundary, probably representing the ILM and the IS/OS junction. The ILM and the IS/OS junction are raised and sectioned transversely in the shape of a crown.

forms an irregular circle connected to the temporal part of the posterior pole. Given the concave shape of the retina, a horizontal section will involve multiple retinal layers, from the ILM and the RNFL to the more interior layers of the photoreceptors, the RPE, and the choroid **(Figures 2-4)**.

We continue to explore the full utility of 3D studies of retinal pathology, but already we recognize how our understanding of certain diseases can be improved. We can now view vitreal and vitreoretinal changes and identify the resulting distortion in the macula. We also can see the characteristics of tangential or posterior traction, such as cellophane maculopathy and macular pucker with centripetal traction, either constant or intermittent **(Figures 11A-B)**.

In cystoid macular edema, the RPE-fit enables us to measure pseudocysts and evaluate their topography to determine if they are circular or irregular within the fovea. The C-scan allows us to determine the number, dimensions, and topography of pseudocysts within a macular or lamellar hole at any thickness **(Figures 10A-B)**. There are, in fact, differences which must be examined in depth.

Serous detachments of the RPE reveal that, according to the etiology, the borders are more or less regular, smooth or irregular, rounded or polyoblate. Thus, we can evaluate the thickness of the borders of the detachment **(Figures 12A-D)**.

"EN FACE" ONE CLICK MODE RTVUE 100 SD-OCT

To make simpler and faster acquisition and use of "en face" images, RTVue 100 software has recently proposed the "en face one click mode" (Lumbroso-vue) that permits to obtain in a single move five scans: four "en face" images relative to the most clinically important frontal sections, and a cross line scan.

The first en face scan is taken at retinal surface level and shows retina vitreous interface alterations, the second is placed deeper in retina and shows eventually diffuse edema, cystoid edema and exudates. The third en face scan is parallel to retinal pigment epithelium and cuts through drusen and to retinal pigment epithelium detachments. The fourth scan is in the choroid, parallel to retinal pigment epithelium at level of Haller vascular layer to show choroid condition.

The OCT cross line scan shows the exact level in the retina of the four frontal scans.

Thus in an immediate and easy way OCT user will get instantaneously the four "en face" images most clinically useful to fine-tune diagnosis, and will know their exact position in relation to retina and choroid layers.

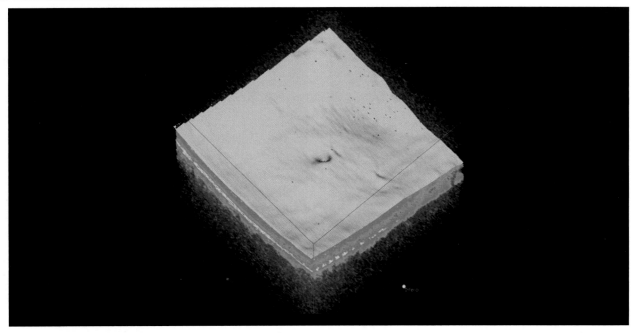

FIGURE 10A. LAMELLAR HOLE.
This is a 3-D representation of the retinal cube, showing the ILM.

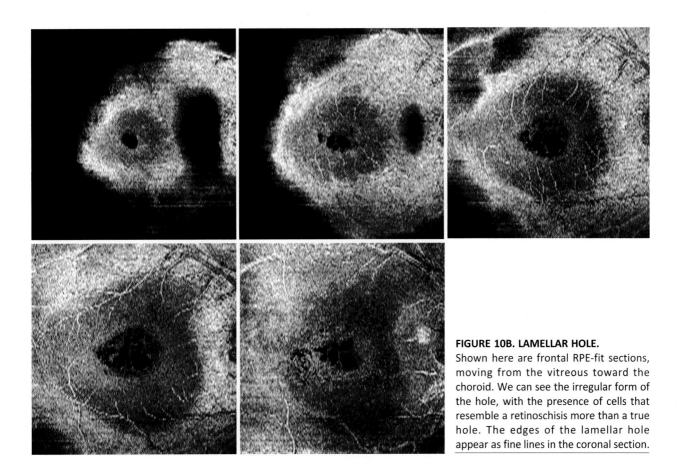

FIGURE 10B. LAMELLAR HOLE.
Shown here are frontal RPE-fit sections, moving from the vitreous toward the choroid. We can see the irregular form of the hole, with the presence of cells that resemble a retinoschisis more than a true hole. The edges of the lamellar hole appear as fine lines in the coronal section.

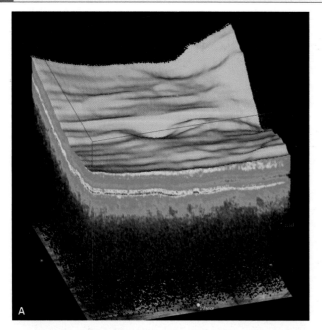
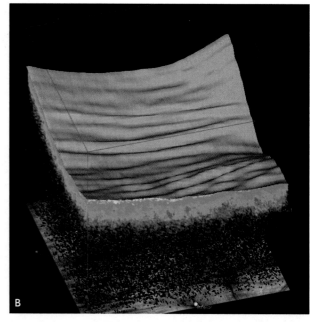

FIGURES 11A-B. CHOROIDAL FOLDS IN AN EYE WITH HYPOTONY.
A: Internal limiting membrane. Parallel horizontal retinal folds are visible.
B: Three-dimensional retinal cube with total removal of the internal retina, showing RPE layer with choroidal folds.

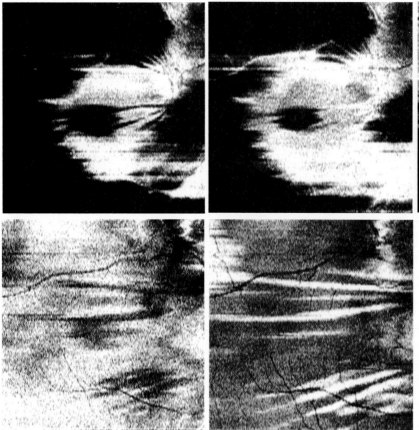

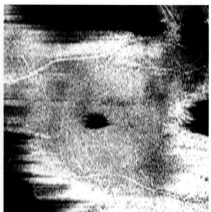

FIGURE 11C. PARALLEL FRONTAL SECTIONS ADAPTED TO THE RPE CURVATURE.
These sections are not flat, but adapted to the curvature of the RPE/choriocapillaris by the RPE-fit function. The frontal sections begin at the surface and terminate at the RPE, showing the parallelism of the folds.

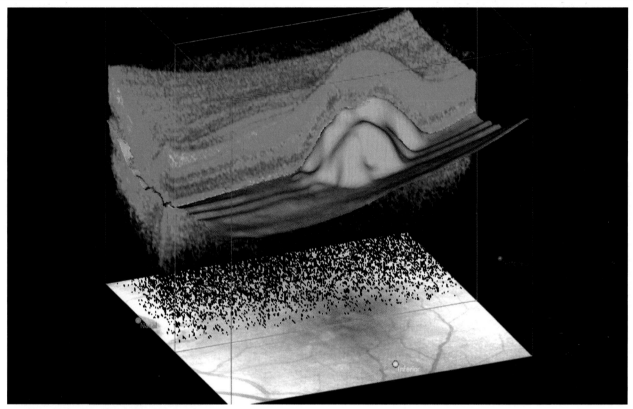

FIGURE 12A. RPE DETACHMENT IN AMD PATIENT.
The retinal cube has been sectioned to show the RPE detachment.

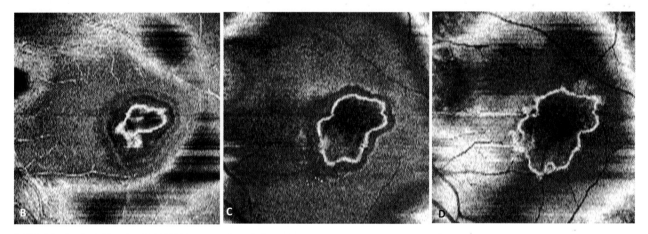

FIGURES 12B-D. RPE DETACHMENT IN AMD PATIENT. FRONTAL SECTIONS ADAPTED TO THE RPE CURVATURE.
These images correspond to the eye shown in Figure 12A. The serous detachment has been sectioned, starting from the retinal surface and moving toward the choroid.
Figure 12B, a superficial section, shows the thickened, irregular boundary, with small spikes penetrating the interior of the detachment.
Figure 12C, a deeper section, shows the boundary irregularly thickened in some areas and thinner in others. Inside this, a hyporeflective area represents a small serous detachment of the epithelium.
Figure 12D, a section that passes radially through the RPE, showing the greater irregularity of the base of the detachment.

Chapter 5

Retinal Topography with Spectral Domain OCT

Spectral domain OCT technology has significantly advanced the study of retinal topography.

Topography scans obtained with time domain optical coherence tomography (OCT) were produced using two modes, which have some limitations. The first mode was based on the acquisition of six radial B-scans centered on a fixation point. The software drew two segmentation lines on the OCT scan, which traced the retinal structure at the vitreoretinal interface and the retinal pigment epithelium (RPE). Time domain instruments successively calculated the thickness between these six radial scans, interpolating the space between the scans. These calculations were accurate near the center, but sensitivity decreased toward the periphery of the scan as the spacing between the radial lines decreased. Another limitation of this procedure was that the junction of the radial scans sometimes was misaligned because its location depends on the stability of the patient's fixation and degree of cooperation.

In comparison, spectral domain OCT technology produces scans with better resolution and in less time,[1,2] thus it is possible to apply a topographical acquisition algorithm that is more sensitive and more reliably repeatable. Using a series of close horizontal scans, it is possible to construct a three-dimensional (3-D) cube of the retina with resolution that is directly proportional to the acquisition time for each B-scan.

SPECTRAL DOMAIN PROTOCOLS

The Cirrus™ HD-OCT has two commonly used protocols for retinal imaging, 512×128 and 200x200. The latter is faster and gives good resolution for most pathologies. The 512×128 protocol analyzes 128 horizontal scans at high resolution (512 A-scans per B-scan). This enables the identification of the retinal infrastructure in far greater detail than can be achieved with time domain technology. The RPE/choriocapillaris complex, for example, is not comprised of two hyperreflective bands, but rather the external llimiting membrane, the junction of the internal and external segments of the photoreceptors (IS/OS junction), a hyporeflective band, and the complex consisting of the RPE and Bruch's/choriocapillaris membrane. The software and other calculation functions ensure the correct positioning of the external markers for analysis of the retinal map.

From the retinal cube, it is possible to extrapolate a thickness map with reference between the ILM and the RPE and the 3-D profile of the ILM and the RPE taken individually.

Using a more precise measurement in the context of the retinal map, the ETDRS grid is superimposed on the fundus image, automatically and precisely centered on the fovea. Average thickness values for each sector are indicated numerically and by a color

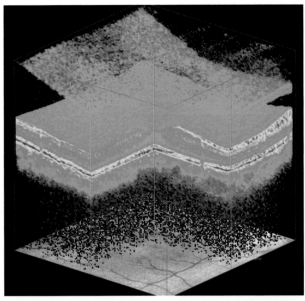

FIGURE 1. RETINAL CUBE.
Part of the tissue is removed to show the cross section of retinal section.

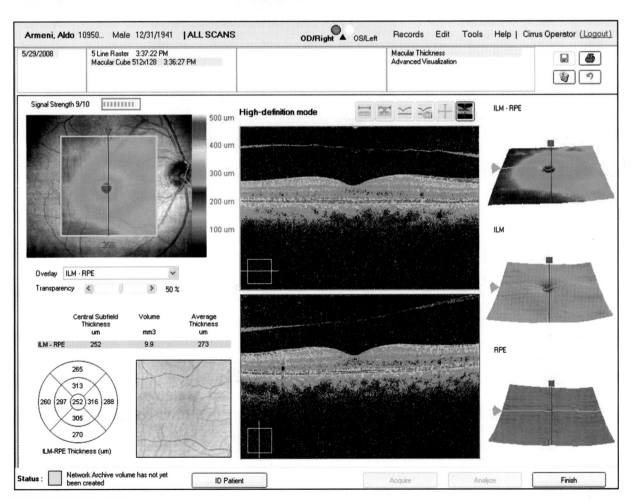

FIGURE 2. NORMAL MAP.
The screen for the retinal map provides numerous data. A false-color representation of the macular area is subdivided into sectors, showing average thickness for each sector. Near this are high-resolution horizontal and vertical scans and a display of the OCT fundus image. On the right of the screen are three layer maps: the ILM-RPE, displaying the retinal thickness in three dimensions, and the ILM and the RPE separately to facilitate evaluation of changes in the corresponding layer.

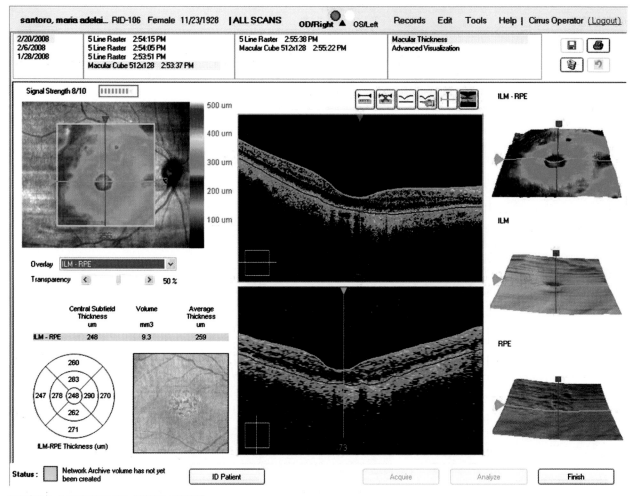

FIGURE 3. PARTIALLY ATROPHIED RETINA.
On the right of the screen, three maps correspond to three distinct layers. The ILM-RPE, display the retinal thickness in three dimensions. The ILM layer and the RPE layer facilitate evaluation of changes.

scale. The color map has variable transparency when superimposed on the fundus image.

To complete the topographical study, there is the option of extracting the horizontal and vertical B-scans that cross any point on the map to evaluate a lesion that causes topographical alterations. In this case, the horizontal scan is one of those used by the OCT to produce the map, while the vertical scan is reconstructed from the horizontal A-scans **(Figures 1-3).** In the 200x200 protocol, the vertical and horizontal scans have equal resolution. In the 512x128 protocol, the vertical scan has lower resolution.

REFERENCES

1. Gupta V, Gupta P, Singh R, Dogra MR, Gupta A. Spectral-domain Cirrus high-definition optical coherence tomography is better than time-domain Stratus optical coherence tomography for evaluation of macular pathologic features in uveitis. *Am J Ophthalmol* 2008;146:626-627.
2. Leung CK, Cheung CY, Weinreb RN, Lee G, Lin D, Pang CP, Lam DS. Comparison of macular thickness measurements between time domain and spectral domain optical coherence tomography. *Invest Ophthalmol Vis Sci.* 2008;49:4893-4897.

Chapter 6

Spectral Domain OCT for the Study and Management of Glaucoma

Spectral domain OCT provides important data to guide clinical decision-making.

Optical coherence tomography (OCT) contributes to our ability to manage glaucoma by providing important qualitative and quantitative data. It enables us to study the morphology and morphometry of the optic disc and the peripapillary nerve fibers. Even using first-generation OCT, the direct measurement of the thickness of the retinal nerve fiber layer (RNFL) enables *in vivo* visualization of retinal sections. Numerous studies have shown a correspondence between OCT measurements and histological measurements.[1-3] For this reason, clinicians are studying RNFL thickness more frequently to aid in early diagnosis of glaucoma and to obtain an accurate assessment of disease progression.

CIRRUS™ HD-OCT SPECTRAL DOMAIN TECHNOLOGY FOR THE STUDY OF GLAUCOMA

The Cirrus™ HD-OCT spectral domain technology is further advancing the study of glaucoma. It employs a simple, easy-to-use system, which allows us to precisely capture and clearly display information about the peripapillary area and the RNFL.

OPTIC DISC SCAN

The Cirrus™ HD-OCT scan of the optic disc captures a 6x6-mm cube, which is formed from 200 A-scans for each of 200 B-scans. The area within the 6x6-mm area is segmented for analysis.

From this cube of data, the machine automatically identifies the center of the disc and creates a 3.46-mm calculation circle around the disc. The RNFL thickness along this peripapillary circle is analyzed and compared to normative data. Even if the scan is not centered on the optic disc, the RNFL circle analysis will be automatically centered, assuring precise registration and excellent repeatability.

RNFL NORMATIVE DATABASE

The RNFL normative database helps us identify areas of clinical interest by comparing patients' RNFL thickness measurements with age-matched normal subjects. The normative data are displayed whenever a glaucoma analysis is performed for a patient over 18 years of age.

The RNFL normative database uses color to indicate the normal distribution percentiles among individuals of the same age, as follows:

- *Red*: The lowest 1% of measurements fall within the red zone. These readings are considered outside normal limits, i.e. pathological.
- *Yellow*: The lowest 5% of measurements fall within or under the yellow zone and are considered suspects.

■ *Green*: 90% of all measurements fall within the green zone and are considered normal.

The highest 5% of measurements fall within the white area.

When interpreting the normative data, we must remember that for each measurement, 1 in 20 normal eyes (5%) will fall below the green zone.

SIGNAL STRENGTH

The Signal Strength Value, which applies to the entire scan, ranges from 0 to 10, with 10 being maximum signal strength. Values less than 5 indicate the signal strength is below the acceptable threshold.

However, since with some patients, a high signal strength may not be possible, the operator/clinician should review the scan and analysis, to determine if it is acceptable.

FUNDUS IMAGE

The scanning laser ophthalmoscope (SLO) fundus image with OCT fundus image overlay is displayed at the top of the RNFL analysis screen or printout. The location of the calculation circle for the temporal, superior, nasal, inferior, temporal (TSNIT) analysis is illustrated in red. The operator can adjust the circle for analysis after scan acquisition, but this usually is not necessary because the automatic centering is accurate. The B-scan image shown is the calculation circle extracted from the cube of data and flattened to a TSNIT orientation.

RNFL THICKNESS MAP

The RNFL thickness map is based on data calculated over the entire cube. Using a color scale similar to a topographical map — cool colors represent thinner areas and warm colors represent thicker areas — it shows RNFL thickness at each point within the 6x6-mm area. The maps exclude the optic disc, which is displayed in dark blue. The color code expresses the thickness from zero (blue) to 350 micrometers (white), illustrating where defects exist.

Deviation Map

The deviation map compares the patient's RNFL thickness versus normative data. Data points that are outside normal limits are shown in red and yellow as described above.

Average Thickness Values

The RNFL thickness along the TSNIT calculation circle is also illustrated numerically in chart format. The average thickness for all points along the calculation circle is shown for both eyes. Average thickness is also shown for each quadrant and for the clock hours. In each of these charts, the patient's values are compared to normative data. The data table calls out symmetry, which is also compared to normative data.

TSNIT THICKNESS PROFILES

The TSNIT profiles show RNFL thickness at each position along the peripapillary analysis circle and compares these measurements with a normative database. They are color-coded (white, green, yellow, red) for comparison with the normative RNFL data for subjects of the same age.

A graph showing RNFL thickness for both eyes highlights asymmetry **(Figures 1–3).**

SUMMARY OF RESULTS

The results of the glaucoma analysis are presented in a table for easy at-a-glance assessment. In the first row at the top are the images of the fundus and the B-scan of the nerve fibers relative to the peripapillary circle. In the second row are the relative maps of the thickness of the nerve fibers, and next to them, the relative maps of the difference between the normal thickness and the thickness found in the examination (deviation map).

In the third row are the circles showing the thickness of the nerve fibers in the quadrants. In the fourth row, the thickness of the fibers is shown in microns in a colored table, where we can easily see if the curve is within the green (normal) range, the yellow (suspect) range, or the red, which is clearly pathological. Data for the right eye are shown on the left, and for the left eye on the right.

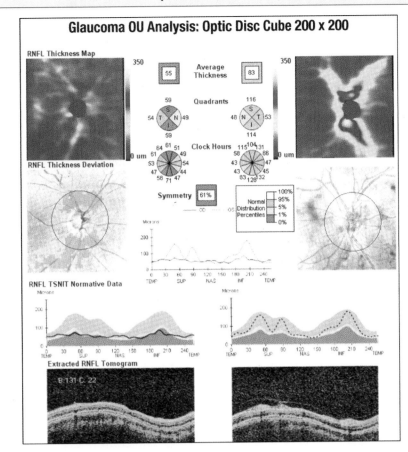

Glaucoma OU Analysis: Optic Disc Cube 200 x 200

FIGURE 1. NORMAL EYE.

This map shows a comparison of a patient's RNFL thickness with the normative database. In this mode, it is easy and intuitive to see the extent and location of nerve fiber defects.

The display shows both eyes, facilitating comparisons when only one eye is affected by the pathology. The area within the deviation map is displayed in a false-color scale, using warm colors (red and yellow) to show the extent and location of defects; the absence of color represents normal thickness.

In the fourth row, a graphic combines the curves of the RNFL thickness of the right eye and those of the left eye, showing their difference **(Figures 1–3)**.

IMPORTANT DIAGNOSTIC TOOL

The Cirrus™ HD-OCT enables us to obtain and display numerous data related to glaucomatous damage in a clear and obvious manner. We must remember, however that the study of glaucoma is complex, and the information provided by a single instrument, however precise, is not sufficient to diagnose more difficult cases. We must base our diagnoses on all of our clinical examinations, including perimetry.

For Glaucoma, Guided Progression Analysis (GPA) compares RNFL thickness measurements from the Optic Disc Cube scan over time and determines if statistically significant change has occurred. The results show event analysis, trend analysis and a quantified rate of change.

OPTOVUE SPECTRAL DOMAIN TECHNOLOGY FOR THE STUDY OF GLAUCOMA

RTVUE 100 GLAUCOMA SCAN PROTOCOLS

To study glaucoma RTVue uses four scan modalities. It can use the same protocols as the other devices do, but also another protocol that assesses the Ganglion Cell Complex in the macular region. This is a different diagnostic tool; it offers the possibility of ganglion cell layer evaluation, and allows confronting to data normal for age and ethnicity.

1. **Optic disc scan protocol.** Optic disc limits are calculated from a 6x6 mm cube, formed by 101 lines. Disc boundary that is automatically drawn by the software using the 3D Disc scan. It is used as baseline and to identify rim and disc vessels.

2. **Retinal nerve fiber layer scan protocol** is used to assess nerve fiber thickness. The RNFL scan pattern completes four circular scans in 0.16

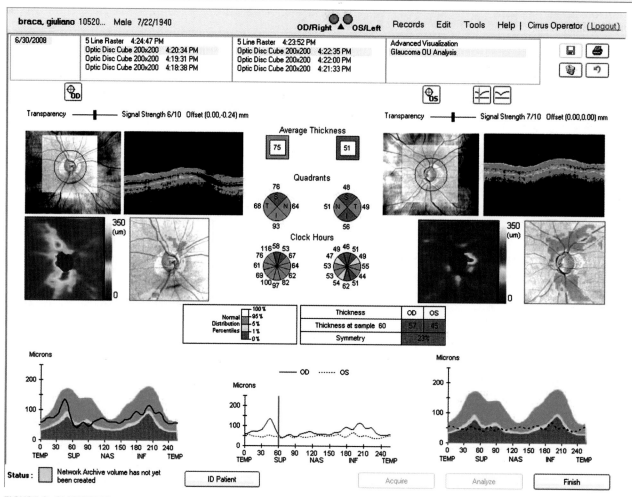

FIGURE 2. GLAUCOMA.

When compared with the normative database, this patient's RNFL thickness is almost entirely outside normal limits. Values for the right eye are almost entirely in the green zone, while values for the left eye are within the yellow and red pathological zones. The deviation map uses warm colors (red and yellow) to show the extent of the deficit in the left eye. These RNFL defects must be compared with the visual fields as shown in Figure 3.

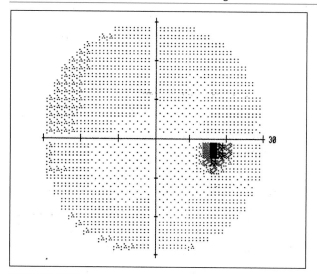
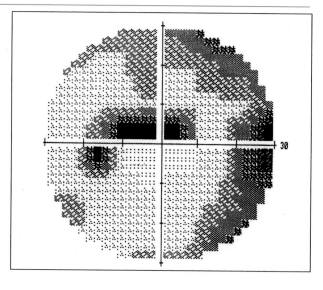

FIGURE 3. VISUAL FIELDS OF BOTH EYES RELATIVE TO FIGURE 2.

The visual field defects correspond with the RNFL deviations shown by the Cirrus™ HD-OCT scan.

seconds at a diameter of 3.45 mm, targeted around the optic nerve head. These four scans are averaged and the result is compared with the normative range parameters. Retinal nerve fiber layer thickness profile in the ONH is the thickness of RNFL at a *calculated* 3.45 mm diameter around the *center* of the disc not the center of the scan. Eventually the de-centering of the disc will not affect the measurement.

3. **Optic nerve head map**. This protocol completes 13 circular scans at a diameter of 1.3 to 4.9, targeted around the optic nerve head, and 9 radial scans. They delimit the space between pigment epithelium and optic nerve head. The device calculates automatically the *center* of the disc, not the center of the scan. The same center point will be automatically used for the progression maps. Optic Nerve Head map gives important disc morphology information: Disc and Cup Areas, Cup/Disc Ratio, RNFL 3.45 and NFL thickness map from disc margin up to 2 mm radius from the center of disc.

4. **The GCC (Ganglion cell complex) map.** Nerve fibers layer, ganglion cells layer and inner plexiform layer form the Ganglion Cell Complex in the macular region. The scan applies 12 vertical lines 7 mm long and one horizontal line 7 mm long. They are placed at 0.5 mm interval and centered 1 mm temporal to fovea to include the largest possible extent of ganglion cells. It can display the thickness map and deviation from normal of the Inner Retina.[4]

The **Deviation map** shows the deviation from normality for age and ethnicity as presented by normative database.

The **Significance map** reports the patient findings compared to normal as presented by normative database. It uses red, yellow and green color to note the changes during the follow up. It indicates the degree of significance, or the statistical probability that the deviation is significant as related to matched normal. More simply it shows how important is the difference with normality.

Focal Loss Volume (FLV) is a parameter that provides a quantitative measure for the amount of significant GCC loss. FLV is the total sum of significant GCC loss (in volume) divided by the map area. It seems that FLV is the most accurate parameter to differentiate normal from glaucomatous eyes, being better than the average GCC thickness parameter.

RTVue study of the Ganglion Cell Complex in the macular region is an important diagnostic tool; it offers a unique possibility of assessment of ganglion cell layer status, and allows confronting to data normal for age and ethnicity.

NORMATIVE DATABASE

The RTVue database of 600 eyes (US) and 1000 eyes (international) is the largest OCT database. It includes data for both **retina** (*edema and ischemia*) and **glaucoma** (*Optic Disc, ppRNFL, NFL to 4 mm and Ganglion Cell Complex*). It helps us comparing patients measurements with age-matched normal subjects. The RNFL normative database uses color to indicate the normal distribution among individuals of the same age. Red: indicate that readings are pathological, outside normal limits. Yellow: indicates borderline readings, they fall inside the yellow zone and are considered suspects. Green measurements are normal.

The normative database parameters are segmented by three factors:
1. **Age segmentation** (Retina and glaucoma maps)
2. **Optic disc size** (only in conjunction with the ONH scan)
3. **Ethnic segmentation**: African descendant, Chinese, Japanese, Caucasian, Hispanic, Indian, Other/combined (this is the default selection if no Ethnicity is selected by the user).

The normative database is used to inform it a particular patient's results fall within the parameters of the "normal" population range for their age and ethnic group. The RTVue normative database was collected at 10 clinical sites around the world. The RTVue software allows to annotate the ethnic origin when entering patient data.

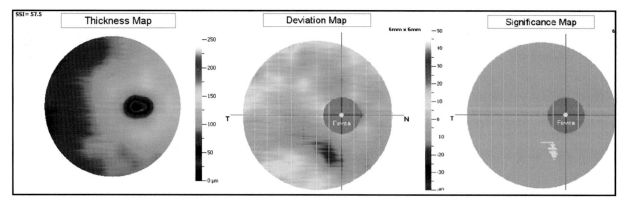

FIGURE 4: GCC, NORMAL EYE. GCC MAP, DEVIATION MAP, SIGNIFICANCE MAP IN NORMAL EYE. RTVUE-100.

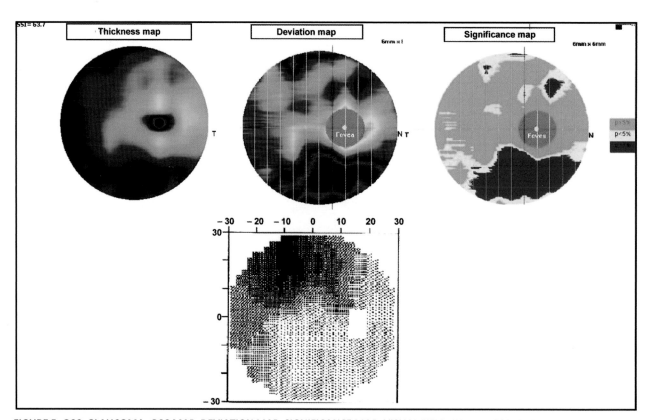

FIGURE 5: GCC, GLAUCOMA. GCC MAP, DEVIATION MAP, SIGNIFICANCE MAP, VISUAL FIELD IN GLAUCOMATOUS EYE. RTVUE-100.
When compared with the database, this patient's Ganglion Cell Complex thickness is outside normal limits in the inferior retina. Values for inferior retina are in the blue and black zone for the deviation map. The right eye is almost entirely in the green zone, while values within the yellow and red pathological zones for the significance map. The visual field defects correspond with the GCC deviations shown by the RTVue OCT scan.

It is important to know that normative database comparisons are based on statistics only and that it is possible to find normal persons outside normal database range. We must remember that 5% of normal eyes will fall in the yellow or even red zone. To reduce the risk of diagnosis errors we cannot rely only on database: it should only one of many clinical information.

GLAUCOMA FOLLOW-UP

RTVue Progression analysis compares RNFL thickness measurements and Ganglion cell complex maps over time and determines if statistically significant change has occurred. The rate of change is quantified.[5]

REFERENCES

1. Abbott CJ, McBrien NA, Grünert U, Pianta MJ. Relationship of the optical coherence tomography signal to underlying retinal histology in the tree shrew (Tupaia belangeri). *Invest Ophthalmol Vis Sci.* 2009;50:214-223.
2. Chen TC, Cense B, Miller JW, et al. Histologic correlation of *in vivo* optical coherence tomography images of the human retina. *Am J Ophthalmol.* 2006;141:1165-1168.
3. Gloesmann M, Hermann B, Schubert C, Sattmann H, Ahnelt PK, Drexler W. Histologic correlation of pig retina radial stratification with ultra high-resolution optical coherence tomography. *Invest Ophthalmol Vis Sci.* 2003;44:1696-1703.
4. Lindsey S Folio, Gadi Wollstein, Hiroshi Ishikawa, Larry Kagemann, Joel S. Schuman. Diagnosis of glaucomatous optic Neuropathy in Imaging the Eye from front to back with RTVue Fourier-domain optical coherence tomography, David Huang, Jay S. Duker, James G. Fujimoto, Bruno Lumbroso, Joel S. Schuman, Robert N. Weinreb, Slack Inc. 2010
5. Gianmarco Vizzeri, Linda M. Zangwill, Robert N. Weinreb. Detection of glaucomatous progression using spectral-domain optical coherence tomography, in Imaging the Eye from front to back with RTVue Fourier-domain optical coherence tomography, David Huang, Jay S. Duker, James G. Fujimoto, Bruno Lumbroso, Joel S. Schuman, Robert N. Weinreb, Slack Inc. 2010

PART TWO
Clinical Reference Cases

INTRODUCTION

In Part 2 of this handbook, we present reference cases and examples of the data that can be obtained via spectral domain optical coherence tomography. These cases are from our clinical observations in which areas of hyperreflectivity and hyporeflectivity are identified, studied, and associated with various syndromes.

The cases presented first in this section are more frequently encountered. They are followed by more uncommon and complex cases.

CONTENTS

Vitreous and Pathologies of the Vitreoretinal Interface

VITREOUS OPACITY

Opacities of the vitreous are most often associated with vitreous hemorrhage and posterior vitreous detachment. In synchysis scintillans **(Figure 1)**, which can occur after trauma, hemorrhage, and inflammation, the vitreous liquefies, and thick crystalline deposits of cholesterol are present. In asteroid hyalosis **(Figure 2)**, spherical bodies like snowballs of unknown etiology appear in the vitreous.

The syndromes of the vitreoretinal interface vary in severity from simple preretinal membrane to vitreoretinal traction and macular pucker.

VITREOUS TRACTION

In cases of more consistent vitreous traction, a band of hyperreflective vitreous fluid can be seen, resulting from retinal adhesions at one or more points. In these cases, the retinal profile is markedly altered, with a localized increase in retinal thickness and reduced intraretinal reflectivity, at times surrounding a single point of traction, indicated by intraretinal edema **(Figure 3)**.

PRERETINAL AND EPIRETINAL MEMBRANE, CELLOPHANE MACULOPATHY

Membranes can be adherent or detached at various points, causing retinal folds. Optical coherence tomography may show weak reflectivity along the retinal surface, without evidence of changes in thickness or intraretinal reflectivity **(Figures 4, 5, 6)**.

MACULAR PUCKER

An epiretinal membrane (ERM) may appear as a hyperreflective band adhering to the internal retinal surface, with no indication that the retina has separated or that the internal retinal surface has split. A consistent increase in reflectivity and extension of the retinal surface is usually seen. Increased macular thickness with a loss of the foveal depression, accompanied by a somewhat consistent homogeneous and diffuse reduction in intraretinal reflectivity usually indicate macular edema, which may present with a cystoid aspect **(Figure 7)**.

TABLE 1: CHANGES IN THE VITREORETINAL INTERFACE
• Macular pucker
• Anteroposterior traction
• Macular hole and pseudohole
• Syndromes of the interface in diabetic retinopathy

TABLE 2: TYPES OF PRERETINAL AND EPIRETINAL MEMBRANES
• Minimal and translucent
• Dense, with a shadowing effect
• Detached
• Adherent
• Macular pucker

FULL-THICKNESS MACULAR HOLE

A full-thickness macular hole presents as an absence of foveal neuroretinal tissue. The margins of the hole are thickened and may be slightly detached. Intraretinal reflectivity is reduced because of perilesional cystoid edema. The foveal retinal operculum always presents in front of the hole with a somewhat hyper-reflective aspect.

With SD-OCT, we can study the vitreoretinal interface and evaluate the risk of macular holes forming in a patient's other eye based on the presence or absence of traction. Partial detachment of the vitreous, with adherence on the foveal periphery and loss of the normal foveal depression often will signal the potential for a hole. Total detachment of the vitreous impedes the formation of holes.

The C-scan crosses a full-thickness macular hole and shows a perfectly circular aspect of the hole section. Data obtained from the C-scan are more complete than those obtained using other methods.

The C-scan can be used to evaluate the semicircular form and dimensions of the hole, but above all, it precisely shows the form and internal location around the hole of the cystoid macular edema (CME) cells.

It appears that the retinal opercula are connected not only to the superficial retina, but also to the internal limiting membrane (ILM). Three-dimensional (3-D) imaging of the macula enables us to measure the dimensions and surface of macular holes, particularly when they are irregular.

LAMELLAR HOLE

In partial-thickness macular holes, we can see a somewhat consistent reduction in foveal retinal thickness, owing to the disappearance of the internal retinal layers. The external layers, in particular the external nuclear layer (ENL), the ELM, and the junction between the internal and external segments of the photoreceptors (IS/OS junction), are well-preserved. This explains why visual acuity is retained.

The cross section shows a rounded but slightly irregular hole, and an adjacent cell of cystoid edema (Figures 8A-C).

TABLE 3: TOPOGRAPHY OF PRERETINAL AND EPIRETINAL MEMBRANES

- Localized at the macular center
- Decentered
- Extend through the posterior pole

CHARACTERISTICS OF TRACTION
- Tangential: macular pucker
- Centripetal
- Anteroposterior with possible macular hole

OUTCOMES OF VITREORETINAL TRACTION
- Retinal thickening
- Diffuse edema
- Cystoid edema
- Lamellar hole
- Retinal hole
- Retinal fold
- Hemorrhage
- Attenuated blood vessels
- Tractional retinal detachment
- Retinal tears

TABLE 4: GASS'S CLASSIFICATION OF MACULAR HOLES

Stage 1: Diminution and disappearance of the foveal depression and presence of a retinal fissure or a cyst under the fovea. It is often possible to discern tangential or horizontal traction exerted by the posterior hyaloid of the retinal surface.

Stage 2: The intraretinal cyst has developed, greatly thinning the operculum, which remains in part but is still adherent.

Stage 3: Full-thickness hole. The operculum is generally, but not always, visible in front of the hole, and retinal edema is noticeable at the margins.

Stage 4: Full-thickness hole, with the presence of cystoid edema in the retinal tissue; the margins of the hole appear rounded with minimal detachment.

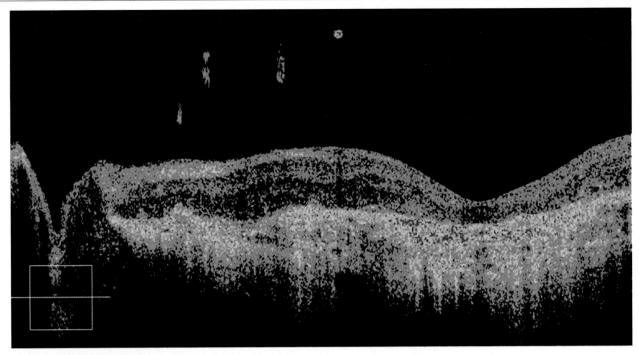

FIGURE 1. SYNCHYSIS SCINTILLANS.
In this eye affected by macular degeneration, small opacities are visible in the vitreous.

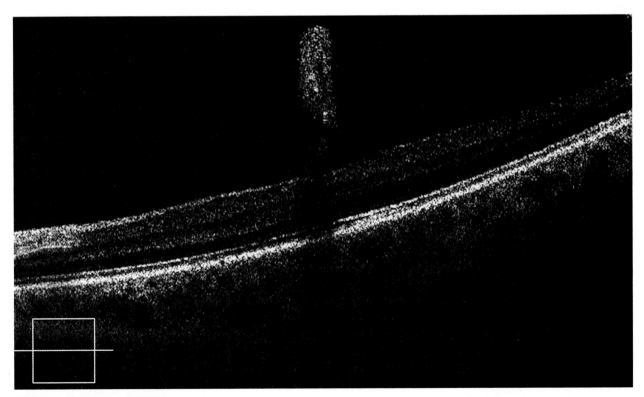

FIGURE 2. PRERETINAL OPACITY.
A thick, snowball-like preretinal opacity is present in the vitreous a few microns from the retina. This opacity is bound to the retina by fine membranes and forms a shadow on the posterior layers.

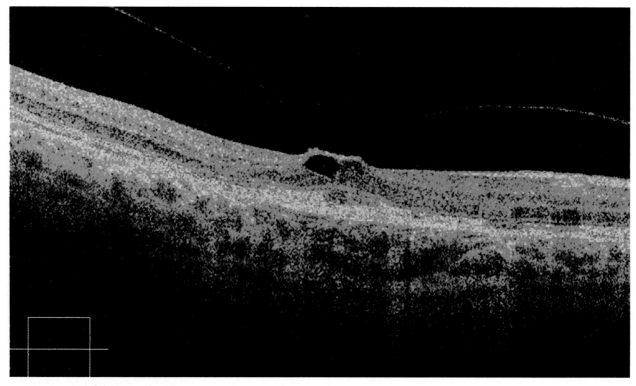

FIGURE 3. VITREORETINAL TRACTION.
The retinal surface at the fovea is altered by marked traction exerted by the vitreous membrane on the fovea. Under the retinal surface is an optically blank, irregular cavity. Diffuse retinal edema is also noted.

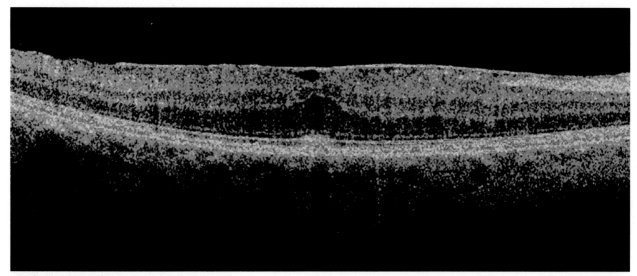

FIGURE 4. ADHERENT ERM – RETINAL EDEMA.
The B-scan shows a hyperreflective, partially detached ERM. There is diffuse retinal edema with a marked increase in thickness at the fovea, where the profile is altered with a convex course. The ELM and the IS/OS junction are normal.

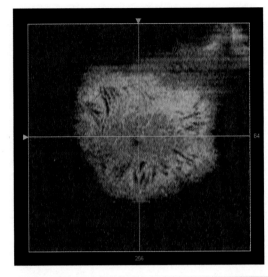

FIGURE 5. ADHERENT ERM – RETINAL EDEMA – FRONTAL SECTIONS ADAPTED TO THE RPE CURVATURE.
This C-scan shows a convex section of the retina in the more internal layers. The scan shows minimal retinal folds formed by the tangential traction exerted by the ERM.

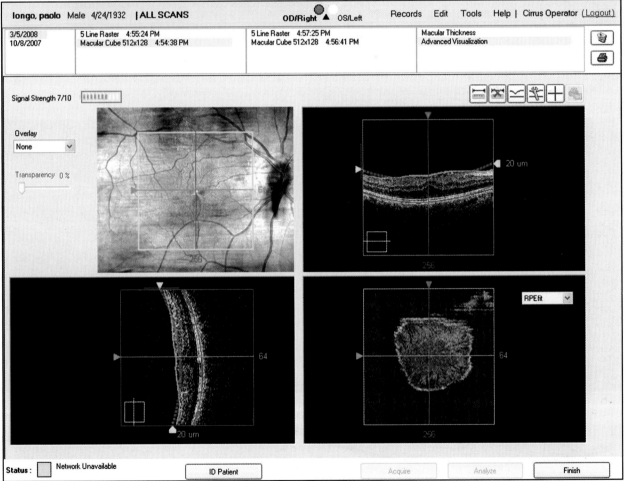

FIGURE 6. ADHERENT ERM- RETINAL EDEMA.
The retinal section (C-scan) of the underside of the membrane highlights the traction exerted on it and on the retinal fold.

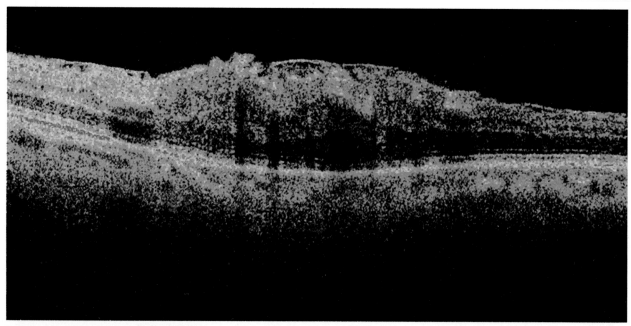

FIGURE 7. B-SCAN OF MACULAR PUCKER.
The scan shows a significantly altered retinal profile. The retina is convex, and the foveal depression is absent; the ERM is thick and partially adherent, while at certain points, splits between the membrane and the retina are apparent. The retinal thickness is increased by diffuse edema.

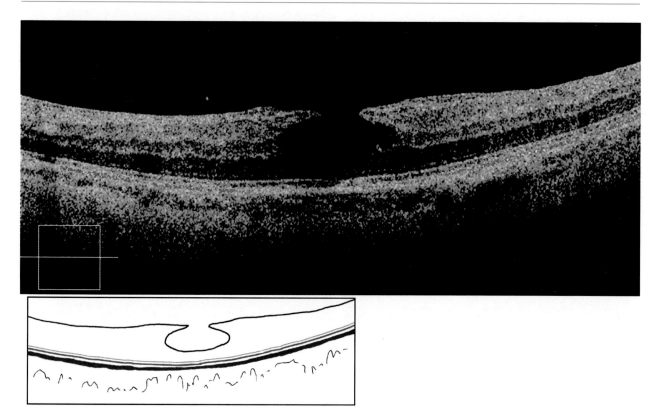

FIGURE 8A. B-SCAN OF LAMELLAR HOLE.
The scan shows the absence of the internal layers of the retina at the fovea, while the more external layers, the external nuclear membrane, the ELM, and the photoreceptors are preserved. This explains why visual acuity is preserved (20/30). The loss is less apparent along the internal layers of the retina in comparison with the layers below.

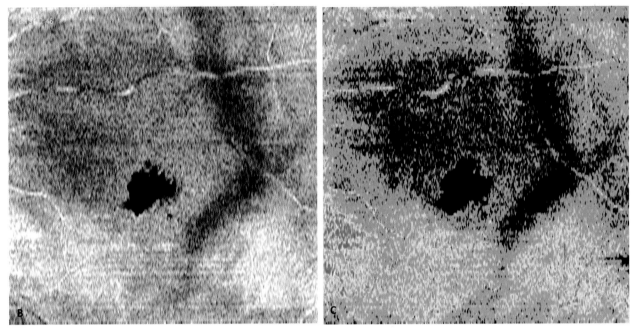

FIGURES 8B- C. LAMELLAR HOLE.
Frontal section adapted to the RPE curvature in black and white and color. The lamellar hole seen from the front exhibits an angular and irregular shape, very different from a full-thickness hole, which usually presents a regular rounded form

Macular Degeneration

Age-related macular degeneration (AMD) is either atrophic or exudative. Atrophic AMD is more prevalent than exudative forms with neovascular membranes. Exudative or "wet" AMD may involve intraretinal retinal angiomatous proliferation (RAP) or anastomoses and polypoidal angiomatosis choroidopathy. Optical coherence tomography plays an important role in guiding treatment decisions.

EXUDATIVE AMD– NEOVASCULAR MEMBRANES

Neovascular membranes appear as one or more masses with irregular, nonhomogeneous reflectivity. They are usually slightly hyperreflective but with more reflective points. It is often difficult to see the neovascular vessels themselves. What can be seen easily is the fibrosity and irregularity of the retinal pigment epithelium (RPE), which appears irregular and thickened.

MEMBRANE LOCATION

In classic neovascularization, illustrated in **Figure 1**, the OCT examination usually shows a hyper-reflective mass that extends above the RPE, raising the neuroretina **(Figures 2A, 2B)**. Retinal edema and small serous detachments of the neuroretina are visible. When neovascular membrane is present, numerous hyperreflective dots are seen frequently at the ENL and the IS/OS junction.

Classic neovascular membranes may be located above the RPE but, at times, they form a body with the distorted RPE and penetrate the thickness of the retina.

Occult neovascular membranes, in general, are located between the RPE and Bruch's membrane. They can cast a shadow on the posterior layers **(Figures 3-4)**.

In more advanced cases, the RPE and Bruch's membrane are distorted or disrupted, and the neovascular vessels penetrate the retina. At this level, the line corresponding to the junction between the internal and external segments of the photoreceptors generally disappears. There is a marked decrease in the thickness of the layer of the nuclei of the photoreceptors (the ENL).

If there is a detachment, the RPE and classic or occult membranes are generally located at the margins of the RPE detachment. When neovascular vessels seem to be in the center of the RPE detachment, this is generally an intraretinal anastomosis.

Small hyperreflective points are found within the neovascularization. In cases of anastomosis, there is always localized dissociation of the deeper layers.

SIGNS ASSOCIATED WITH ACTIVE NEOVASCULARIZATION

Retinal edema, at times cystic, and somewhat sizable serous detachments of the neuroretina are usually present in areas of active neovascular membrane. The high resolution of SD-OCT allows precise imaging of minute areas of intraretinal or subretinal fluid. Small hyperreflective points near the neovascularization may be signs of inflammation **(Figure 8)**.

SEROUS RPE DETACHMENTS

It is important to study the content of a serous RPE detachment to determine if it is vascularized or fibrotic. In fibrovascular RPE detachments, there is

TABLE 1: SIGNS ASSOCIATED WITH ACTIVE NEOVASCULARIZATION

- Retinal edema
- Serous retinal detachment
- Hyperreflective points near the neovascularization

marked hyperreflectivity, and the serous detachment is partially organized **(Figures 5-7)**.

ATROPHIC MACULAR DEGENERATION

In atrophic macular degeneration, the more prevalent form of AMD, the choriocapillaris and the choroid are involved, with marked scleroses of the principal blood vessels. Using OCT, we can observe progressive atrophy of the RPE and the retinal layers, especially the external membrane. There is a markes decrease in retinal thickness due to membranes in the ENL, with changes in the ELM and the IS/OS junction, extending outside the atrophic area.

A marked increase in the reflectivity of the RPE can be noted, due to the atrophy and especially the reduced absorption of light by the altered retinal tissues **(Figure 9)**. The retinal map precisely highlights the boundaries of the atrophic area.

Autofluorescence plays a significant role in tracking the progression of atrophic macular degeneration. It enables us to evaluate the functionality of the retina and can show the extent of the atrophy. Autofluorescence also allows observation of foveal retention.

PSEUDOVITELLIFORM MACULAR DEGENERATION

Pseudovitelliform macular degeneration in adults is a dominant autosomal genetic condition that progresses slowly from the vitelliform stage to the pseudohypopion stage and finally to the atrophic stage. **Figures 10 and 11** show the pseudohypopion stage, with an opaque yellow-orange subretinal deposit and a central retinal detachment. There is a dense, hyperreflective, nodular formation, probably lipofuscin, at the fovea. The overlying retina is thinned.

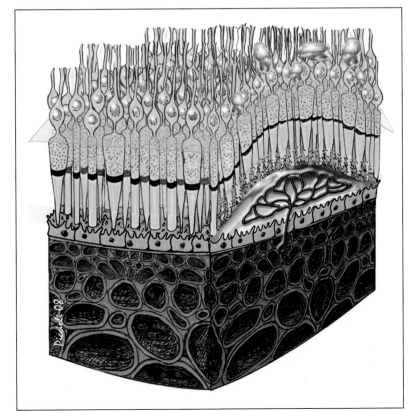

FIGURE 1. CLASSIC NEOVASCULAR MEMBRANE IN AMD WITH SEROUS DETACHMENT OF THE NEURORETINA AND DAMAGE TO PHOTO-RECEPTORS.
This illustration represents a classic neovascular membrane. These membranes develop on top of the RPE after having traversed Bruch's membrane and the epithelium. This may be observed before the serous detachment of the neuroepithelium, which is visible when neovascularization is active and the altered photoreceptors are in contact with the neovascularization.

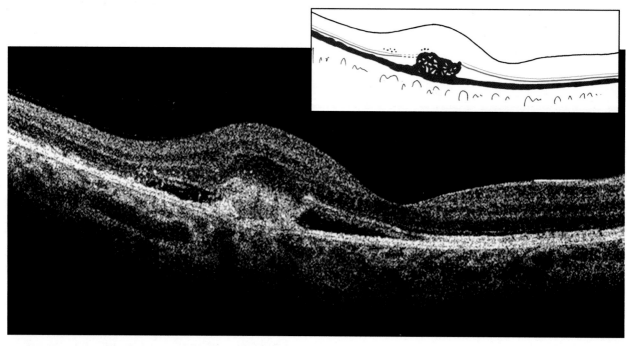

FIGURE 2A. B-SCAN OF CLASSIC NEOVASCULAR MEMBRANE.

The retina is deformed by the neovascular membrane, which is forming a localized detachment of the retina. This classic membrane forms a hyperreflective mass with an irregular and nonhomogeneous shape located in the posterior pole. Above the lesion, small cells of incipient cystoid edema and small hyperreflective points in the deep retina are observed. Around the membrane, between the RPE and the neuroretina, a serous retinal detachment is seen. Incipient cystoid edema, hyperreflective points, and serous retinal detachment are the classic signs that indicate an active membrane. The ELM and the IS/OS junction are easily visible. Bruch's membrane is also interrupted at the area of the neovascularization.

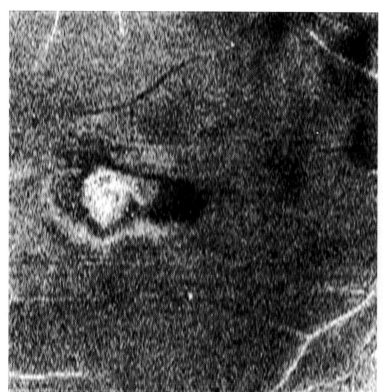

FIGURE 2B. CLASSIC NEOVASCULAR MEMBRANE – FRONTAL SECTION ADAPTED TO THE RPE CONTOUR.

This RPE-fit image, slightly anterior of the RPE, shows a serous detachment of the retina around the neovascularization. At the center of the detachment, an irregular and nonhomogeneous mass of neovascularization is seen.

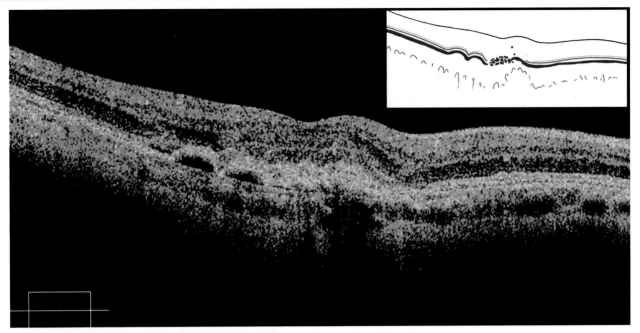

FIGURE 3. OCCULT NEOVASCULAR MEMBRANE IN AMD.

The retina is thickened, with an altered profile. At the RPE level, two small serous detachments with a small detachment of the neuroepithelium are visible. Bruch's membrane is clearly visible. Near it, the RPE is detached and dissociated. Between Bruch's membrane and the dissociated RPE, a nonhomogeneous mass, representing the neovascular membrane is observed. The ELM and the IS/OS junction are altered at the level of the membrane and the RPE detachments.

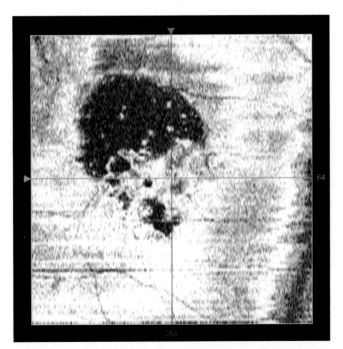

FIGURE 4. OCCULT NEOVASCULAR MEMBRANE IN AMD.

This frontal section is adapted to the RPE contour. The scan passes across the neovascularization, which appears as an irregular and nonhomogeneous mass. Note the two small, round RPE detachments and a small detachment of the neuroepithelium, both with optically blank content.

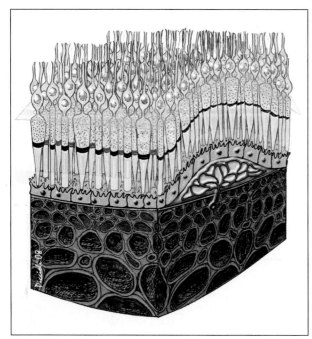

FIGURE 5. NEOVASCULAR MEMBRANE IN AMD – VASCULA- RIZED RPE DETACHMENT.

This illustration shows a serous, vascularized RPE detachment. The neovascularization between Bruch's membrane and the RPE is the beginning of an occult membrane that will result in fragmentation of the RPE.

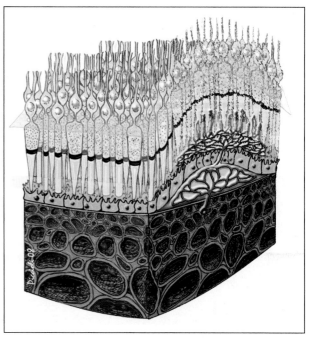

FIGURE 6. NEOVASCULAR MEMBRANE IN AMD.

This illustration represents the progression of the case shown in Figure 5. The neovascular membrane, which originated under the RPE, has developed and led to fragmentation of the epithelium. The neovascular membrane penetrates the neuroretina, crossing the damaged epithelium and inserting itself between the photoreceptors, leading to lesions in the external segments. It then develops toward the nuclear layer (between the cells).

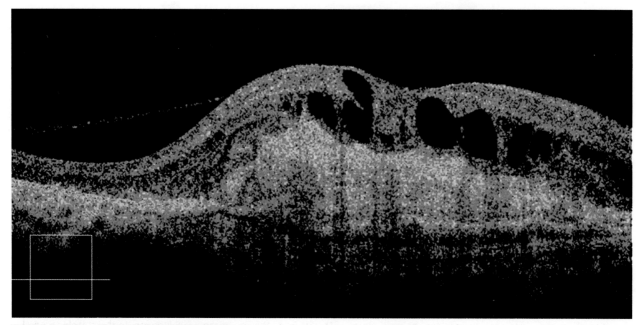

FIGURE 7. AMD – EVOLVED DISCIFORM SHAPE.

The fibrovascular membrane is represented as a significant mass, which fuses with the RPE. This mass is thick and not homogeneous. Above it, the disciform scar of cystoid edema is evident at the retina. The normal layers of the retina cannot be discerned.

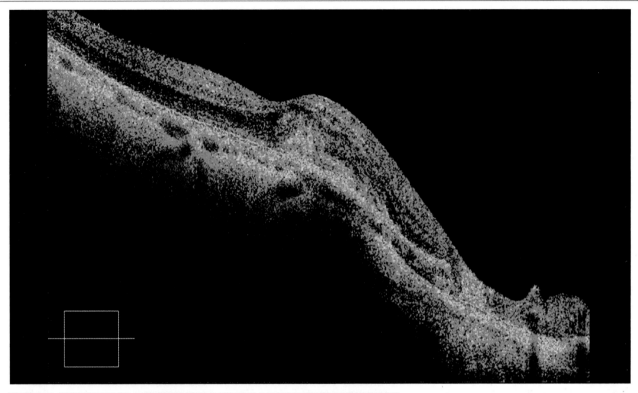

FIGURE 8. NEOVASCULAR MEMBRANE IN A YOUNG PATIENT WITH HIGH MYOPIA.
An ovoid formation in front of the RPE alters the retinal profile. This active fibrovascular formation creates nonhomogeneous reflectivity. The slight retinal edema adjacent to the formation confirms that this is an active membrane. The RPE to the right of the neovascular membrane is clearly altered, almost duplicated.

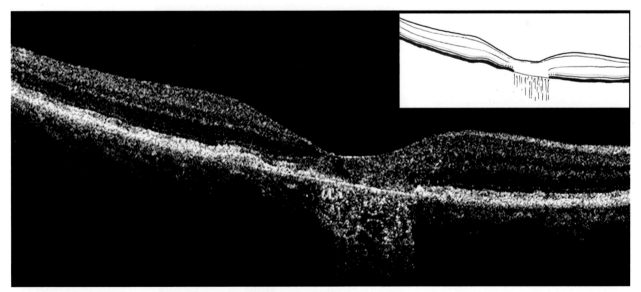

FIGURE 9. B-SCAN OF ATROPHIC MACULAR DEGENERATION – DRUSEN.
The retina is significantly thinned at the posterior pole, with corresponding changes in retinal contour. The marked hyperreflectivity of the choroid at the level of the thinning is due to the absence of retinal and pigment epithelial tissue, permitting light rays to penetrate more deeply into the choroid. In the atrophic area, the retinal layers are altered, with a loss of the normal structure. To the sides of the atrophied area, we can see the persistence of the ELM and the line of the IS/OS junction. In the atrophic area, the RPE is thinned and reduced to Bruch's membrane.

To the left of the retinal atrophy, an undulation in the RPE represents a druse. Under this small undulation, we can see dense, hyperreflective tissue, under which we can see Bruch's membrane, reduced to a subtle line. On top of the undulation, the ELM and the IS/OS junction are normal.

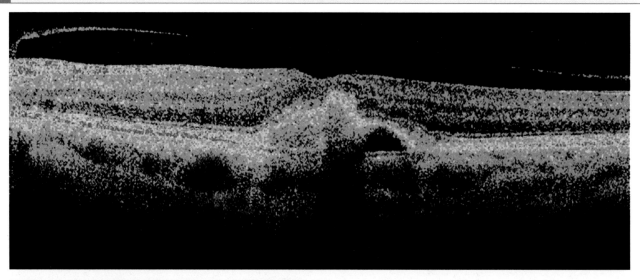

FIGURE 10. PSEUDOVITELLIFORM MACULAR DEGENERATION.

The retinal profile is altered by a hyperreflective mass, forming a body with the RPE (probably lipofuscin). The retina is thinner at the level of this mass. Except for a small area, the ELM and the IS/OS junction are normal at the detachment. Bruch's membrane is visible as is the RPE detachment with optically blank content.

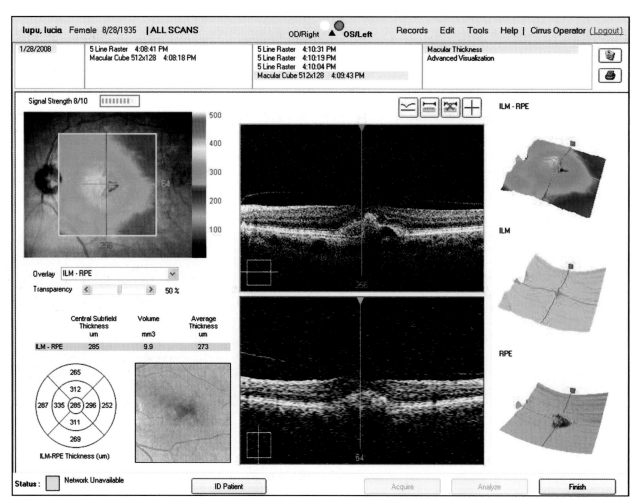

FIGURE 11. PSEUDOVITELLIFORM MACULAR DEGENERATION.

The retinal map shows decreased retinal thickness at the subretinal mass. The 3-D map of the RPE shows the detachment at the lipofuscin deposits.

Diabetic Retinopathy

MACULAR EDEMA IN NONPROLIFE-RATIVE DIABETIC RETINOPATHY

Macular edema is the chief cause of reduced vision in nonproliferative diabetic retinopathy. The SD-OCT examination, which shows retinal sections with nearly histological precision, has enabled further study of diabetic retinopathy. The edema starts with focal edema, progresses to diffuse edema, and then can become cystic. Serous detachment is part of the progression of diabetic edema.

FOCAL EDEMA

Focal edema can be detected with fluorescein angiography or with OCT, which shows a thickened retina. The OCT retinal map is important in cases of focal edema, because it permits better localization to direct treatment. It also helps confirm treatment efficacy.

DIFFUSE EDEMA

Viewed with OCT, the retina with diffuse edema is thickened and shows small, irregular cavities. The areas of low reflectivity are increased and especially evident in the external retinal layers, where diabetic edema is most frequently found. The external plexiform layer shows the most edema. Areas of spongy edema shown on OCT likely represent altered Müller cells. After years of progression of diffuse edema, the irregular microcavities merge, resulting in pseudocysts **(Figures 1A, 1B)**.

EPIRETINAL MEMBRANE

In many cases of retinal edema, OCT enables us to detect an epiretinal membrane (ERM). At times, these are easily differentiated, but sometimes they are merged with the retinal nerve fiber layer (RNFL). This membrane, with its retinal tractions, exacerbates edema and can cause serous detachments. The neuroretina appears thickened, and the foveal depression disappears. In many cases, the tension exerted by the ERM leads to a syndrome of the vitreoretinal interface **(Figures 2-3)**.

CYSTOID MACULAR EDEMA

Persistent retinal edema results in necrosis of the Müller cells, leading to the formation of cystoid cavities in the retina. These cavities start in the external plexiform layer and subsequently penetrate the granular layers and the internal plexiform layer. Advanced cystoid edema permeates the retina, causing residual tissue to atrophy.

It is important to quantify the edema by measuring both volume and thickness of the retina to develop a map of the retinal edema.

TABLE 1: THE ROLE OF OCT IN MANAGING DIABETIC RETINOPATHY
Optical coherence tomography allows us to:
• Investigate causes for decreased visual acuity
• Determine the status of the retina and monitor changes
• Detect the presence of retinal edema, its extent and characteristics
• Quantify edema and measure its volume
• Calculate retinal thickness
• Localize treatment areas by means of retinal topography and C-scan
• Monitor treatment efficacy
• Determine if vitreoretinal surgery is necessary
• Monitor natural history

Optical coherence tomography has become indispensable for detecting and studying diabetic retinopathy in its various stages. In certain cases, it can replace fluorescein angiography, allowing improved detection and quantification of lesions.

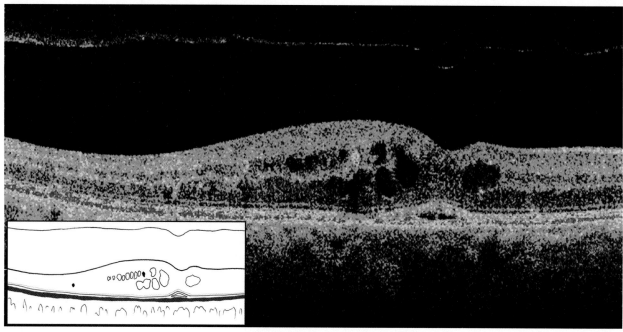

FIGURE 1A. B-SCAN OF NONPROLIFERATIVE DIABETIC RETINOPATHY – INCIPIENT CME.
The hyaloid is detached. The retinal profile is irregular, with deformation of the foveal depression. There are small, optically blank cavities of cystoid edema in the retina, specifically at the INL and the ENL. In place of the fovea, there is a small serous detachment of the neuroretina, which can often be seen in cases of chronic CME. Dense, hyperreflective points due to the exudates of hard lipids are also seen. The ELM and the IS/OS junction are normal in this case.

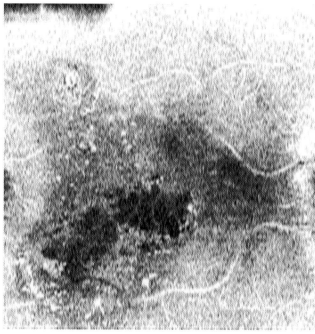

FIGURE 1B. CME IN NONPROLIFERATIVE DIABETIC RETINO-PATHY, FRONTAL SECTION ADAPTED TO THE RPE CONTOUR.
Irregular cells of cystoid edema are clearly visible, especially at the foveal level. Dense formations of hard exudate can be seen.

SEROUS DETACHMENT

Optical coherence tomography has shown that serous detachments are part of the final progression of diabetic edema. A serous retinal detachment with optically blank cavities between the detached retina and the RPE can be seen. A serous detachment can be associated with increased thickness of the detached retina, or the detached retina may appear normal or even atrophied. We have found that serous detachment is frequent and associated mainly with cystoid edema.

QUANTIFICATION

There is a roughly inverse relationship between visual acuity and retinal thickness. As retinal thickness increases, visual acuity decreases with or without the presence of cystoid edema. Measuring the retina's thickness and volume is important for determining prognosis, assessing indications for surgery and monitoring disease progression.

The retinal map is important for localizing focal edema. Measuring retinal thickness allows us to quantify edema, which enables us to track the efficacy of therapy. In our experience, when compared with fluorescein angiography, OCT has demonstrated superior capabilities to aid in the diagnosis of macular edema. It also allows us to distinguish between retinal edema and serous detachment, which cannot be done using fluorescein angiography.

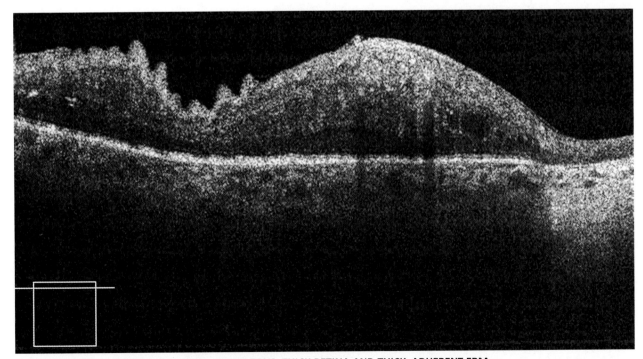

FIGURE 2. DIABETIC RETINOPATHY WITH EDEMATOUS, THICK RETINA AND THICK, ADHERENT ERM.
The retinal profile is irregular. Exudates and cystoid edema are seen in the retina. To the right, corresponding to a laser-treated zone, marked atrophy of the retina is seen, with an increase in reflectivity.

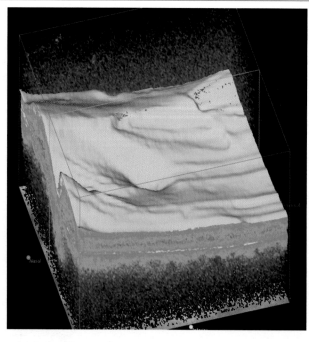

FIGURE 3. DIABETIC RETINOPATHY.
This is a 3-D representation of the retinal cube in Figure 2. The ILM is adherent to the retina, and variations in the retinal thickness follow.

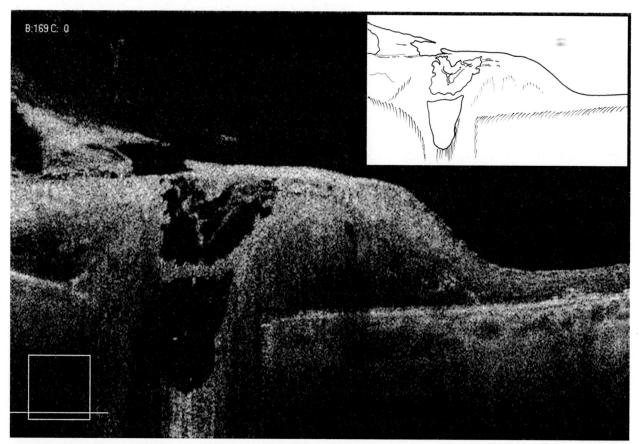

FIGURE 4. PROLIFERATIVE DIABETIC RETINOPATHY – B-SCAN – OPTIC PAPILLA.
Peripapillary neovascular membrane, which is partially regressed after panretinal laser treatment, is seen. The papillary excavation is partially filled with fibrovascular tissue. To the right of the image, an area of retinal atrophy resulting from laser treatment is seen.

CME AFTER CATARACT SURGERY (IRVINE-GASS SYNDROME)

After cataract surgery, visual acuity may become markedly reduced because of CME, which presents as central hyperfluorescence on fluorescein angiography. **Figures 5A and 5B** show a case with numerous intraretinal cysts in the perifoveal area, especially in the internal nuclear layer (INL). The most central cysts of edema occupy the entire thickness of the retina, terminating at the IS/OS junction, which appears altered. The condition usually resolves after treatment.

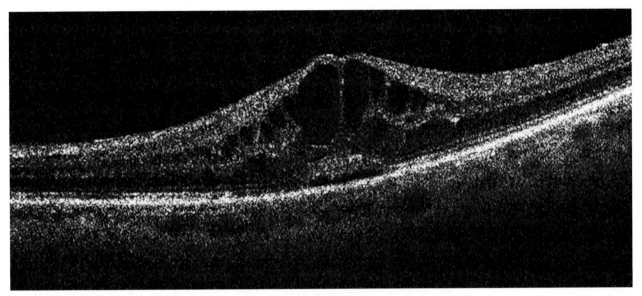

FIGURE 5A. B-SCAN OF CME AFTER CATARACT SURGERY (IRVINE-GASS SYNDROME).
This 82-year-old patient noted decreased visual acuity a few weeks after cataract surgery. The B-scan shows CME involving the INL. We can see optically blank cavities of cystoid edema, mostly in the internal and external nucleus layers. Retinal thickness is greatly increased, while the ELM and the IS/OS junction are well-preserved.

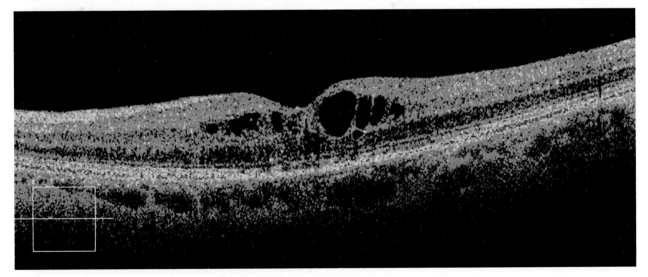

FIGURE 5B. B-SCAN OF CME AFTER CATARACT SURGERY.
This is the fellow eye from the case shown in Figure 5A. CME is also found here, but much less severe than in the other eye.

Vascular Occlusion of the Retina

When an occlusion of the central retinal artery is observed after a few hours, white retinal edema is seen as well as a cherry-red central stain on examination. Optical coherence tomography performed in the first few days allows us to see marked edema, localized in the internal layers: the RNFL, the ganglion layer, the internal plexiform layer and the INL of the bipolar cells. An increase in the reflectivity and thickness of the INL and the RNFL can be observed.

After 15 days, the increased reflectivity and thickness of the INL and RNFL persist, but the reflectivity of the outer retina decreases. After 30 days, the retinal edema has resolved. At that point, a decrease in the thickness of the retina can be seen, with distinct changes, especially of the internal retinal layers. After 6 months, atrophy of the internal retina is observed, with involvement of the photoreceptors **(Figures 2, 3, 6, 7)**.

Vein occlusions can be nonischemic, ischemic, mixed or inflammatory **(Figures 4, 5)**.

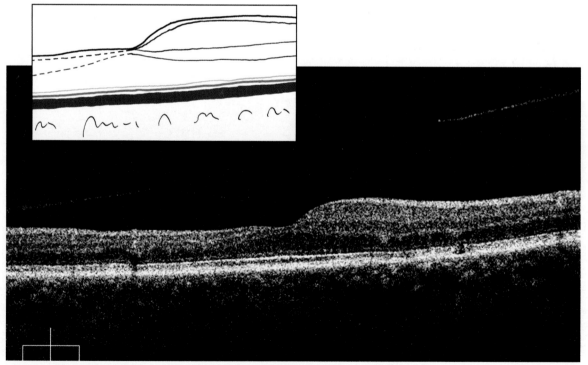

FIGURE 1. 6 MONTHS POST BRANCH RETINAL ARTERY OCCLUSION.
On the right of the B-scan is a normal retina with all layers evident; on the left, an atrophic zone corresponds to the occlusion of the arterial branch. Note that the atrophy almost exclusively involves the internal retinal layers, while the ENL, the ELM, and the IS/OS junction are nearly normal.

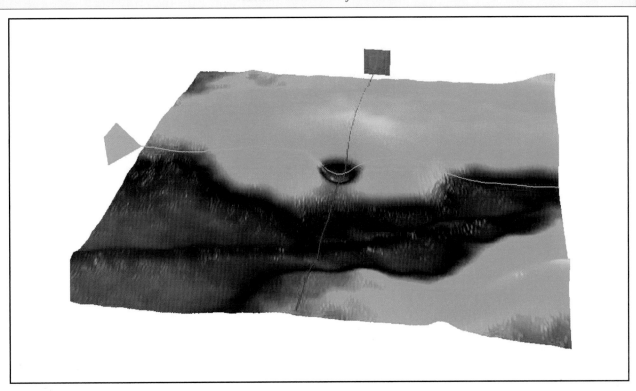

FIGURE 2. 3-D MAP SIX MONTHS POST BRANCH RETINAL ARTERY OCCLUSION.
This 3-D retinal map shows the area of retinal atrophy corresponding to the arterial branch occlusion.

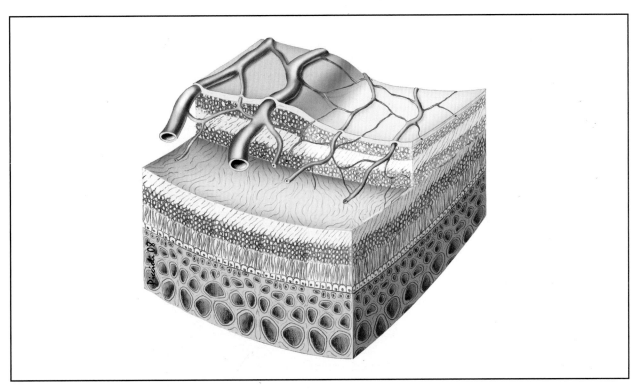

FIGURE 3. SIX MONTHS POST BRANCH RETINAL ARTERY OCCLUSION.
The left part of this illustration shows a normal retina with normal thickness and color, and blood vessels of the usual size. The right half shows atrophy of the internal layers of the retina. The vascular branches are shown very thin to represent their occlusion. The ischemic zone is pale pink with nuclei changes, while the zone of normal perfusion is red.

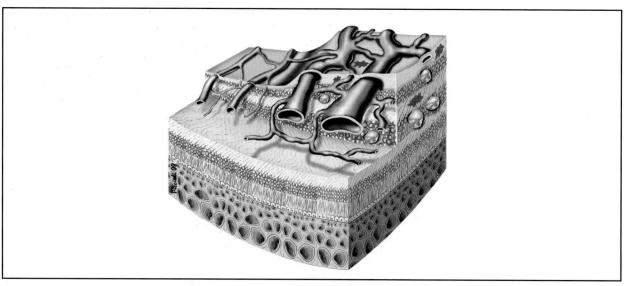

FIGURE 4. BRANCH RETINAL VEIN OCCLUSION.

The left half of the illustration shows a normal retina with blood vessels of normal size. The right half shows thickened retina with dilated and deformed blood vessels. Hemorrhages are shown in the RNFL and the external plexiform layer; edematous cells are shown in the INL and the ganglion layer.

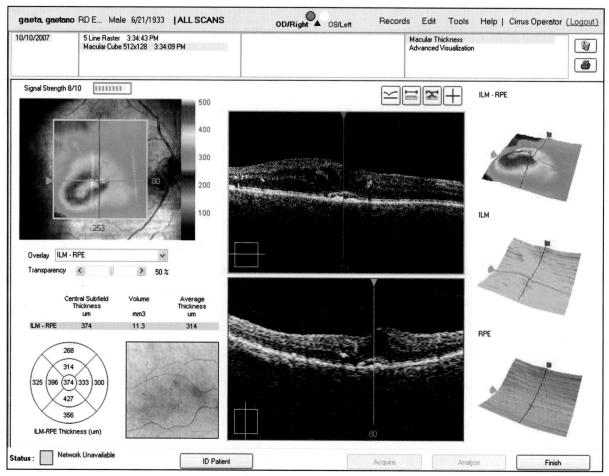

FIGURE 5. RETINAL MAP OF BRANCH RETINAL VEIN OCCLUSION.

Occlusion of a small branch vein is present at the posterior pole near the fovea. Localized edema in the affected branch is evident inferior and temporal of the fovea on the 3-D image, which shows the ILM-RPE thickness.

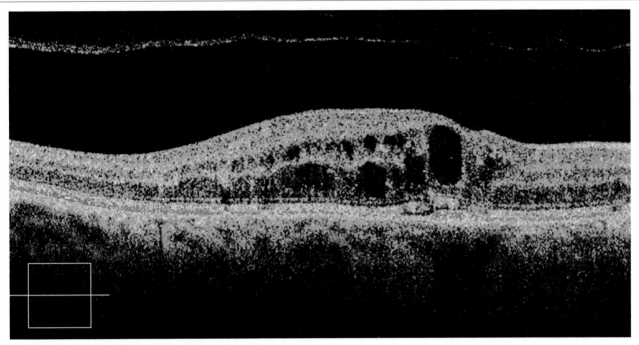

FIGURE 6. B-SCAN OF BRANCH RETINAL VEIN OCCLUSION.

The retinal thickness to the right and left appears normal, while in the center at the fovea, the retina is edematous, thickened with cystoid edema cells. This edema occupies part of the INL with small cysts, while the ENL is involved with larger and more irregular cysts. Toward the fovea, a large edematous cavity occupies the entire thickness of the retina. Exudates are visible between the edematous retina and the normal retina, with a shadow on the posterior layers. The ELM is normal, except at the vascular occlusion.

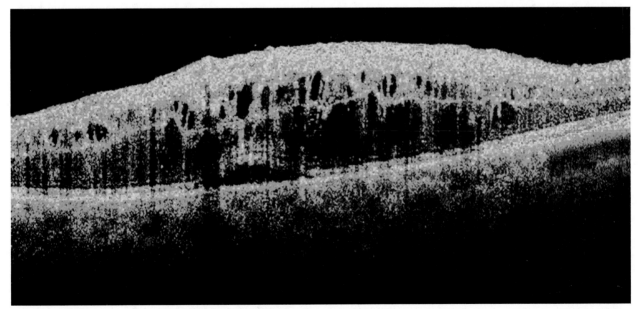

FIGURE 7. B-SCAN OF CENTRAL RETINAL VEIN OCCLUSION.

Marked thickening of the retina with diffuse edema at the RNFL and the ganglion layer is seen. The cells of cystoid edema occupy the entire thickness of the INL. The ENL is distorted by large, irregular cells of edema. These cavities cause alterations to the ELM and the IS/OS junction.

Retinal Epitheliopathy

SEROUS CHORIORETINOPATHY

Central serous chorioretinopathy (CSCR) most commonly occurs in men between 25 and 45 years of age; it is often bilateral and recurrent. Typically, fluorescein angiography reveals a point of diffusion that appears early and increases progressively. In serous RPE detachments, multiple leakage point may be visible where the RPE is detached from Bruch's membrane, forming spaces that fill with fluorescein dye.

In acute CSCR, OCT may reveal a small break in the RPE at the diffusion point inside the serous RPE detachment. From this opening, we may occasionally see reflective material that seems to leak from the choroid toward the interior of the detachment. In cases of acute CSCR, all layers and retinal stripes appear normal in the nondetached retina **(Figure 1)**.

At the serous detachment, either the IS/OS junction or the tips of the photoreceptors are detached, showing a marked reflectivity. The external stripes corresponding to the RPE and Bruch's membrane remain in place. In most eyes with active serous chorioretinopathy, structural changes of the external segment of the photoreceptors are evident. It may be thickened, irregular or have increased reflectivity, with granulations of the internal face of the detachment in the detached area **(Figure 2)**. The IS/OS junction in the detached retina is often irregular in thickness.

CHRONIC EPITHELIOPATHY OR DIFFUSE RETINAL PIGMENT EPITHELIOPATHY

Chronic epitheliopathy usually occurs in people 45 to 69 years of age. It is associated with points of diffusion, dystrophic changes of the RPE and serous RPE detachments. Areas of the RPE may be absent, and areas of gravitational epitheliopathy can be observed. Choroidal neovascularization is common.

In the advanced, chronic form of serous chorioretinopathy, with resolution of the detachments, the ELM is generally visible on OCT, and there is thinning of the ENL associated with changes at the IS/OS junction. The foveal ENL shows increased reflectivity in cases where the serous detachment has resolved. This increased reflectivity of the nuclear layer of the photoreceptors is probably a result of changes to the normal anatomy or formations of fibrous tissue. Other visible changes are retinal thinning at the fovea and, sometimes, true atrophy. The ELM is always visible, allowing evaluation of the changes to the IS/OS junction, which are almost always associated with a thinning of the ENL. The margin of IS/OS junction may be thickened, irregular, or distorted.

Over the course of the natural history or after treatment, a slight thinning of the retina may be seen, with changes to the ELM and the IS/OS junction **(Figures 3A, 3B, 4)**.

TABLE 1: FORMS OF RPE DETACHMENT

Idiopathic detachment
- Simple or multiple

Detachment associated with:
- Acute CSCR (acute serous retinal epitheliopathy)
- Diffuse retinal epitheliopathy or chronic serous chorioretinopathy

Vascularized detachment
- Age-related macular degeneration with subretinal neovascularization
- Retinal angiomatous proliferation
- Polypoidal choroidopathy
- Subretinal neovascularization of other origin

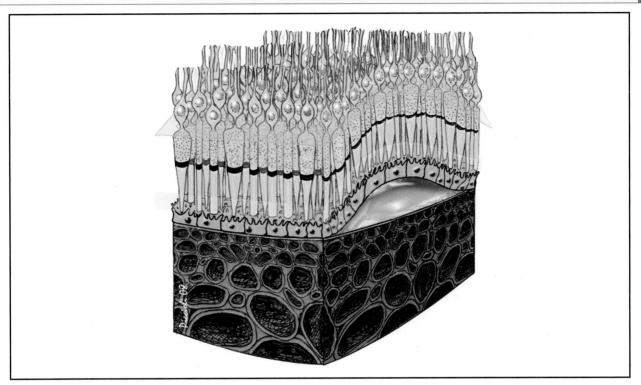

FIGURE 1. SEROUS RPE DETACHMENT IN CSCR.
The RPE has detached from Bruch's membrane, detaching the retina without causing changes to the RPE. The detachment is optically clear, and there is no diffusion of the subretinal fluid.

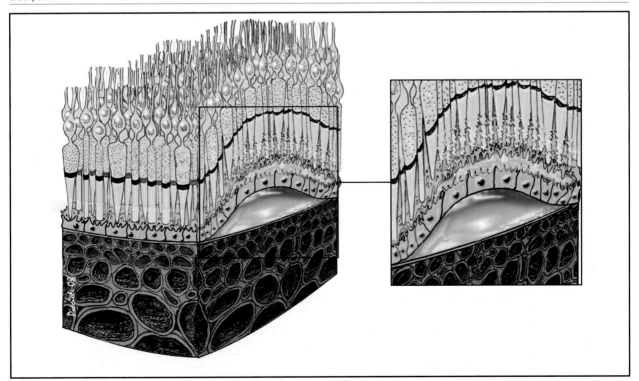

FIGURE 2. RPE DETACHMENT ASSOCIATED WITH SEROUS DETACHMENT OF THE NEUROEPITHELIUM – LESIONS TO THE PHOTORECEPTORS.
In this case of acute CSCR, a leakage point has formed between the cells of the altered RPE, and fluid has diffused beneath the retina, detaching it. Alterations are apparent in the external segment of the photoreceptors. These alterations can be seen when the serous detachment persists for more than a few weeks.

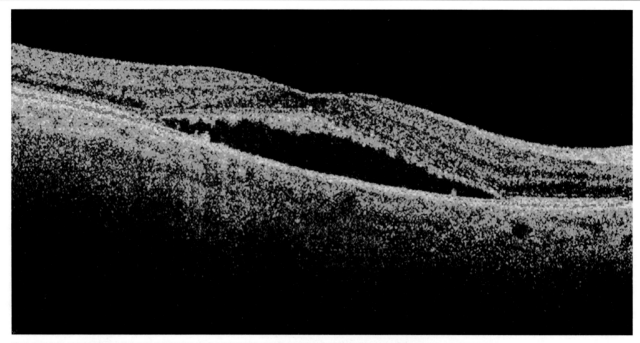

FIGURE 3A. SEROUS DETACHMENT OF THE NEUROEPITHELIUM – LESIONS OF THE PHOTORECEPTORS.
The IS/OS junction and the linear structure corresponding to the tip of the external segment of the photoreceptors lose their clear contours, becoming indistinct and irregular; the layers appear granular and lose integrity.

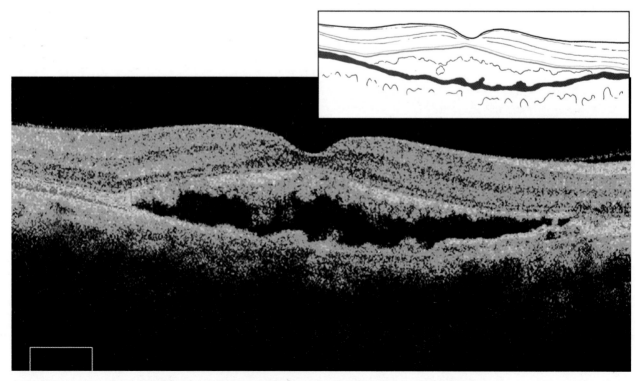

FIGURE 3B. SEROUS DETACHMENT OF THE NEUROEPITHELIUM – LESIONS OF THE PHOTORECEPTORS.
As in Figure 3A, the IS/OS junction and the linear structure corresponding to the external segment of the photoreceptors become indistinct and irregular; the layers become granular and lose integrity. In this case, the changes are more apparent.

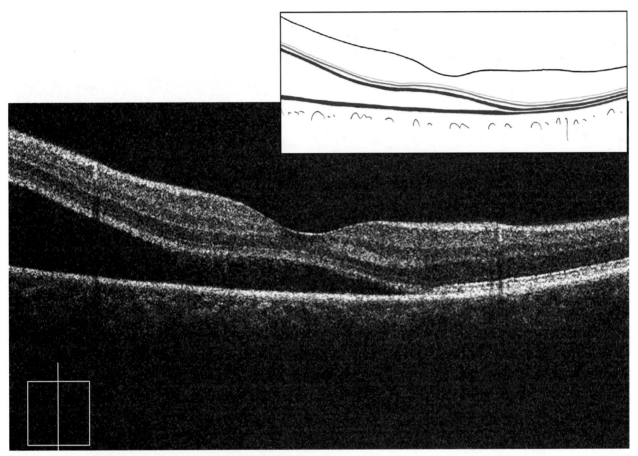

FIGURE 4. SEROUS DETACHMENT OF THE NEUROEPITHELIUM.

This 40-year-old patient complained of worsening vision for more than a year. Fluorescein angiography detected a serous detachment of the retina, with a clear leakage point, away from the fovea.

Spectral domain OCT shows a detachment of the neuroepithelium at the fovea, forming an acute angle with the RPE. The ENL, the ELM, and the IS/OS junction are easily seen. Visual acuity (8/10) is well-preserved.

The RPE appears shaped by two hyperreflective layers separated by a hyporeflective layer in the detachment..

At the detachment, the RPE is divided into two parts: the internal layer follows the detachment and is probably formed by the tip of the photoreceptors; and the RPE remains attached.

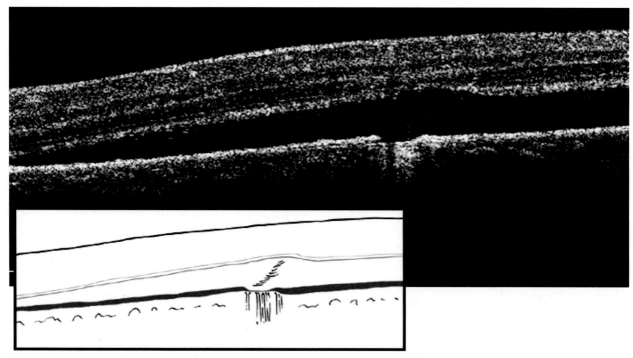

FIGURE 5A. SEROUS DETACHMENT OF THE NEUROEPITHELIUM – POINTS OF DIFFUSION.
In the patient in Figure 4, OCT was performed at the leakage point shown in the fluorescein angiogram below. This diffusion point corresponds to an RPE defect, perhaps reduced to Bruch's membrane. At this level, a slight hyperreflective projection is visible inside the bubble of the detachment, proceeding from the diffusion point. This seems to indicate the diffusion of the fibrin-charged liquid emerging from the choroid.

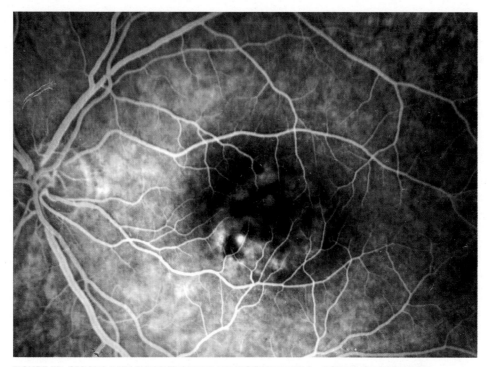

FIGURE 5B. SEROUS DETACHMENT OF THE NEUROEPITHELIUM – POINTS OF DIFFUSION.
On fluorescein angiography, the leakage observed under the macula corresponds to the RPE lesion observed by the OCT B-scan in Figure 5A.

Cysticercosis

We have chosen a case history to illustrate this condition. A 40-year-old man presented with reduced vision for a few weeks. Examination revealed a slight detachment of the retina at the posterior pole under a whitish, ovoid formation in the area between the fovea and the disc **(Figures 1-4)**.

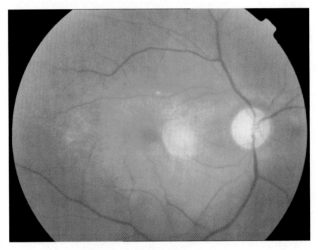

FIGURE 1. SUBRETINAL CYSTICERCOSIS.
This color fundus photo shows the subretinal cyst in the fovea. The cyst is whitish yellow, with a small inferior protrusion, probably the scolex of a tapeworm.

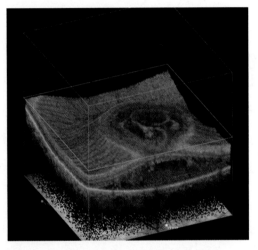

FIGURE 2. C-SCAN OF SUBRETINAL CYSTICERCOSIS.
A frontal C-scan section was performed on the retinal cube. This section shows a rounded mass surrounded by a small serous detachment of the neuroretina.

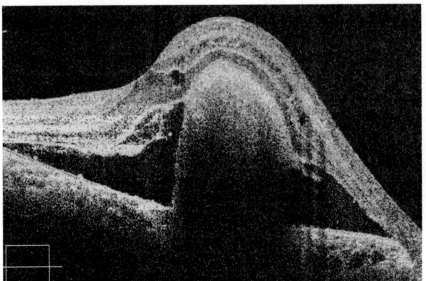

FIGURE 3. B-SCAN OF SUBRETINAL CYSTICERCOSIS.
Spectral domain OCT shows the thickened retina, detached by a subretinal round mass. The retina exhibits cystoid edema at the INL and a few cells of cystoid edema at the ENL. Under the retina a round, cystic formation with hyporeflective contents is visible. The deeper layers of the cysts are not visible, because the light rays do not penetrate the retina and the cyst. There is a circular detachment of the neuroretina.

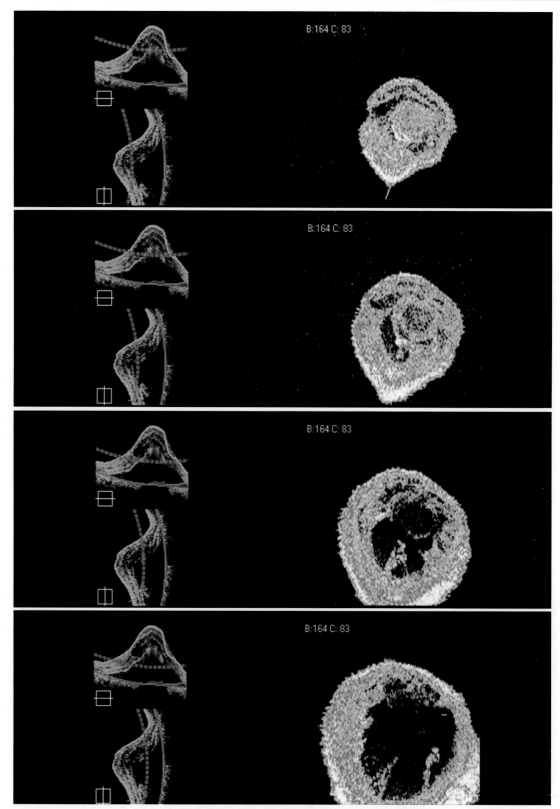

FIGURE 4. SUBRETINAL CYSTICERCOSIS – FRONTAL SECTIONS ADAPTED TO THE RPE CONTOUR.
This series of C-scans show the retina and cyst from top to bottom and the consistent lower reflectivity inside the cyst. It was not possible to detect the scolex. The C-scans show the round cyst and the adherence to the posterior side of the retina. A small hyperreflective mass appears to lie within the lesion.

Vogt-Koyanagi-Harada Syndrome

Vogt-Koyanagi-Harada syndrome is characterized by inflammation of the retina and the choroid in which we can observe anterior and posterior uveitis, along with exudative detachments of the retina with whitish lesions. The serous retinal detachments can merge and cause a significant serous detachment and can involve nearly the entire retina. Disc edema is often associated with this syndrome.

Onset is characterized by worsening of vision, which may be associated with headache and dizziness. As the disease progresses, neovascular membranes and subretinal fibrosis may appear. Headaches and dermatologic disturbances, such as depigmentation and vitiligo, are not always observed. Deafness may also occur.

Fluorescein angiography may demonstrate multiple points of leakage causing a serous detachments of the neuroretina with areas of RPE disturbances **(Figures 1-3)**.

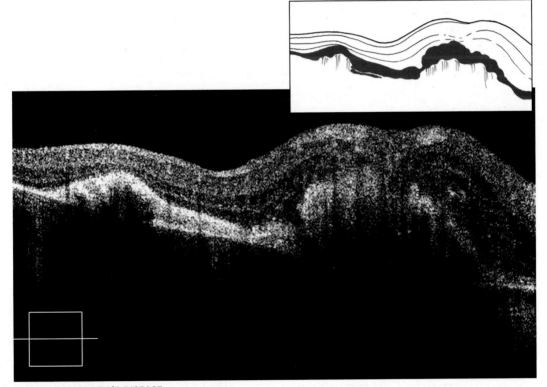

FIGURE 1. B-SCAN OF HARADA'S DISEASE.
The retina is thickened with irregular accumulations of turbid fluid, which are not typical cells of cystoid edema. The RPE is significantly thickened in certain areas. Subretinal exudates may form.

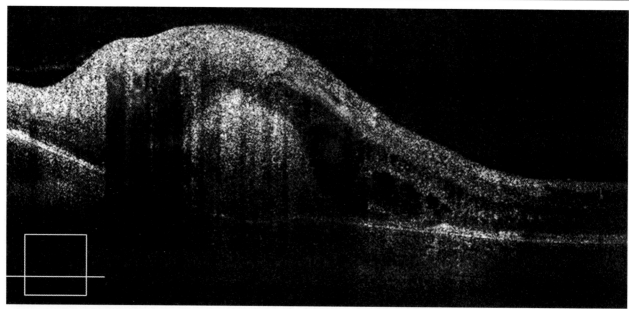

FIGURE 2. HARADA'S DISEASE.

Regression of subretinal fluid is shown. A dense strand of subretinal fibrosis is seen, with a macular detachment. Note irregular accumulations of liquid inside the retina.

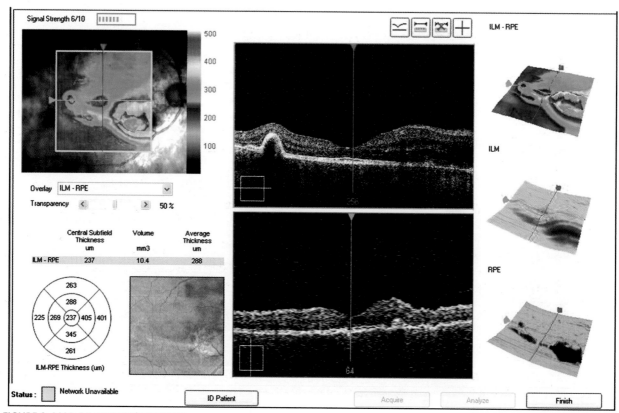

FIGURE 3. MAP OF HARADA'S DISEASE.

The elongated detachment of the retina and the RPE in the inferior peripapillary region subretinal fibrosis, which appeared after 5 years of disease progression.

Complex Cases

The clinical cases presented thus far have ranged from easy to difficult, but all have involved a single pathology. In daily clinical practice, it is not unusual to encounter patients presenting with more complex scenarios with several pathologies. These cases are complicated, requiring analysis of individual pathologies in order to determine the diagnosis that best matches one or more illnesses in a single scan. The following are two particularly complex cases in which a diagnosis based on OCT scans may not be obvious.

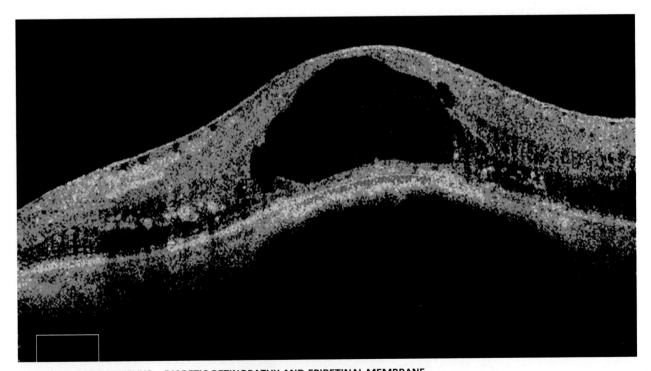

FIGURE 1A. RETINAL NEVUS – DIABETIC RETINOPATHY AND EPIRETINAL MEMBRANE.
This 45-year-old patient has had diabetes for more than 15 years. He presented with pigmented subretinal neoformations.
The B-scan shows a convex deformation of the retina, which is detached by a deep, hyperpigmented mass. The lesion prevents light from penetrating into the choroid. Cystoid edema occupies almost the entire thickness of the retina. Hard lipid exudates are seen in the deep retinal layers. The retinal surface is covered by adherent epiretinal membrane, with some small dehiscences visible.

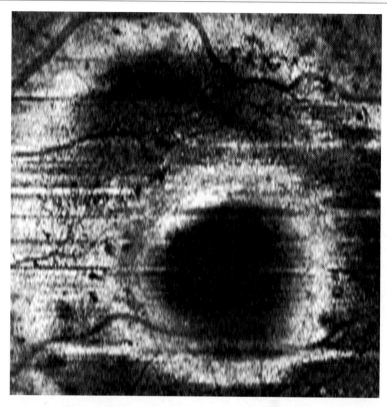

FIGURE 1B. RETINAL NEVUS – DIABETIC RETINOPATHY AND EPIRETINAL MEMBRANE – FRONTAL SCAN ADAPTED TO THE RPE CONTOUR AT THE LEVEL OF THE NEVUS.
The nevus is sectioned transversely, and the scan confirms the presence of a dark, rounded formation circumscribed by a circular hyperreflective boundary under the RPE.

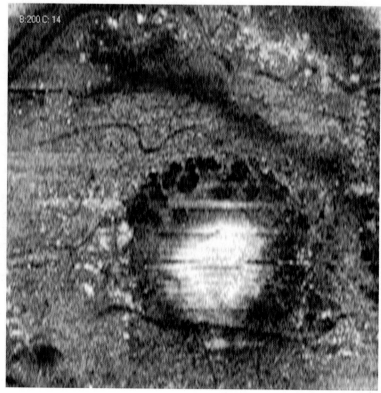

FIGURE 1C. RETINAL NEVUS – DIABETIC RETINO-PATHY AND EPIRETINAL MEMBRANE – FRONTAL SCAN ADAPTED TO THE RPE CONTOUR AT THE LEVEL OF THE RETINA.
The superficial frontal scan traverses the retinal thickness and shows the cystoid edema inside a central hyperreflective area. Hard lipid exudates can be observed in the deep retinal layers.

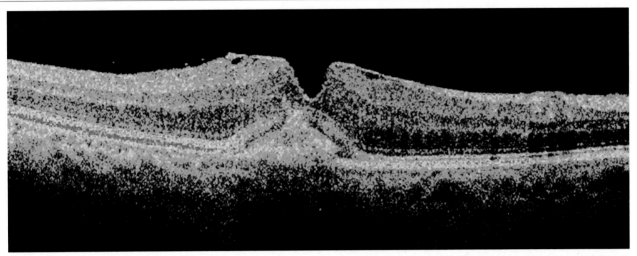

FIGURE 2A. PSEUDOVITELLIFORM MACULAR DEGENERATION – MACULAR PSEUDOHOLE AND SYNDROME OF THE VITREORETINAL INTERFACE.

The B-scan shows that the retinal profile is altered by an adherent preretinal membrane exerting transverse traction on the retina. Also observed is a pseudohole with loss of substance at the internal retinal layers. Accumulated dense, hyperreflective material on and combined with the RPE is found in this eye with pseudovitelliform macular degeneration. The ELM and the IS/OS junction are nearly normal, as reflected in the good visual acuity of 7/10.

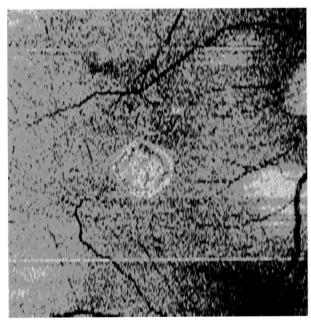

FIGURE 2B. PSEUDOVITELLIFORM MACULAR DEGENERATION – MACULAR PSEUDOHOLE AND SYNDROME OF THE VITREORETINAL INTERFACE – FRONTAL SCAN ADAPTED TO THE RPE CONTOUR.

A dense mass of hyperreflective material can be seen from the pseudovitelliform degeneration. Visible inside is a hyperreflective circle representing the IS/OS junction in frontal section.

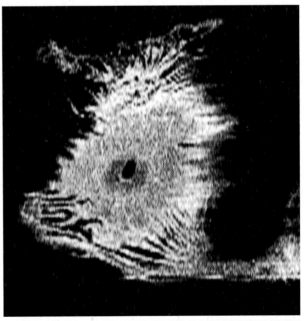

FIGURE 2C. PSEUDOVITELLIFORM MACULAR DEGENERATION – MACULAR PSEUDOHOLE AND SYNDROME OF THE VITREORETINAL INTERFACE – FRONTAL SCAN ADAPTED TO THE RPE CONTOUR.

This scan was performed superficial to the retina. It shows the pseudohole and the superficial retinal folds resulting from the contraction of the ILM.

Spectral Domain OCT: Opening New Vistas in Eye Care

With the new spectral domain optical coherence tomography instruments, we can see structures and obtain information not available with time domain OCT. We can obtain high-resolution images of the posterior pole, showing histological details of the retina. In particular, we can detect with greater precision the ELM, the IS/OS junction, and early damage to the photoreceptors. We are also much more capable of evaluating the external layers of the retina, the ENL, the RPE, Bruch's membrane, and the length of the external segment of the photoreceptors. We can better visualize the choroid and the choriocapillaris. Spectral domain instruments also reconstruct images in three dimensions enabling us to study frontal or cross sections.

Spectral domain OCT is fast and easy to learn and use. It is the ideal instrument for high-level clinical studies, and it can be used for everyday practice, as well.

In conclusion, the **Spectral Domain OCT** represents a great step forward in diagnostic imaging and is appropriate for hospitals and university centers, as well as individual retina specialists, vitreoretinal surgeons and glaucoma specialists.

Index